CARE OF THE
DISABLED URINARY TRACT

CARE OF THE DISABLED URINARY TRACT

PREVENTION OF RENAL DETERIORATION

By

ELLEN NEWMAN, M.T., A.S.C.P., M.S.

Associate Scientist, Microbiologist
Renal Function Laboratory
Department of Physical Medicine and Rehabilitation
University of Minnesota Hospitals, Minneapolis, Minnesota

MARY PRICE, M.S., M.D.

Associate Professor Emeritus
Director, Emeritus Renal Function Laboratory
Clinical Associate Professor
Department of Physical Medicine and Rehabilitation
University of Minnesota
Formerly, Director, Spinal Cord Injury Division
Sister Kenny Institute, Minneapolis, Minnesota

and

JEAN MAGNEY, M.S.

Instructor, Department of Anatomy
Scientific Illustrator
University of Minnesota Medical School, Minneapolis, Minnesota

Foreword by

Elwin E. Fraley, M.D., F.A.C.S.

Professor and Chairman
Department of Urologic Surgery
University of Minnesota Medical School
Chief, Urologic Surgery Service
University of Minnesota Hospitals
Minneapolis, Minnesota

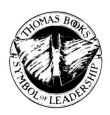

CHARLES C THOMAS • PUBLISHER
Springfield • Illinois • U.S.A.

Published and Distributed Throughout the World by

CHARLES C THOMAS • PUBLISHER
2600 South First Street
Springfield, Illinois 62717

© *1986 by* CHARLES C THOMAS • PUBLISHER

ISBN 0-398-05178-X

Library of Congress Catalog Card Number: 85-17363

With THOMAS BOOKS *careful attention is given to all details of manufacturing and
design. It is the Publisher's desire to present books that are satisfactory as to their physical
qualities and artistic possibilities and appropriate for their particular use.* THOMAS
BOOKS *will be true to those laws of quality that assure a good name and good will.*

Printed in the United States of America
SC-R-3

Library of Congress Cataloging-in-Publication Data

Newman, Ellen.
  Care of the disabled urinary tract.

  Bibliography: p.
  Includes index.
    1. Urinary tract—Diseases—Treatment. 2. Bladder—Diseases—Treatment.
3. Urinary tract infections—Treatment. 4. Chronic diseases—Treatment.
I. Price, Mary, 1917-   . II. Magney, Jean E. III. Title.
RC9005.N49   1986   616.6′06   85-17363
ISBN 0-398-05178-X

This book is dedicated to our many patients who taught us so much.

E.N.
M.P.
J.M.

FOREWORD

The value of meticulous care for patients with a disabled urinary tract has received far too little attention in the past. In fact, if these patients do not receive a high level of treatment from a multidisciplinary team of physicians and other medical personnel, they will lead a miserable life and can look forward to an early death due to kidney failure.

This book represents a splendid effort to present a comprehensive primer on the management of the urinary tract in these patients. It was written by individuals who have devoted a significant part of their professional lives to this subject, and so they share a clear grasp of the problems faced by these patients and an even better understanding of how these patients should be managed. Their approach to treating these patients is grounded on an excellent understanding of anatomy, basic neurophysiology, and infectious disease as it relates to the urinary tract. Thus, the recommendations for management of these patients are, for the most part, logical derivatives from a significant core of fundamental information. Furthermore, the authors advocate the all-important multidisciplinary team approach, which, because of the demanding requirements of these patients, is absolutely essential in offering them optimum care.

In summary, the information presented in this book should serve as an invaluable adjunct to health care personnel who are dealing with patients who have a disabled bladder. It represents one of the most logical and comprehensive treatments of the subject to date and, therefore, is an important contribution to the field. It is also written in a very understandable manner and will therefore serve the needs of physicians as well as other individuals who help care for this group of patients.

Elwin E. Fraley, M.D.

PREFACE

It has long been known that meticulous care of the urinary tract is essential in patients with long-term urinary problems; yet, there is a surprising paucity of specific instructions for accomplishing this goal. This book provides detailed instructions for such care based on eighteen years of research into the renal function of individuals with disabled urinary tracts. It is written for all those who are responsible for patient care: physician, nurse, therapist, counselor, or attendant, as well as the patients and their families.

In 1963 at the University of Minnesota a comprehensive program of patient follow-up was instituted, with special emphasis upon the problems arising from denervation of the bladder. It soon became obvious that the principles of good care for the traumatically induced neurogenic bladder could be applied to other types of neurogenic bladder, including those associated with stroke, multiple sclerosis, diabetes, carcinoma, head injury, acquired anomalies of the spinal cord, congenital defects, and aging.

Consequently, educational programs were devised, first for patients, then for various health professionals such as medical students, residents, practicing physicians, nurses, physical and occupational therapists, psychologists, social workers, and nursing home directors. These programs were sponsored by the Departments of Physical Medicine and Rehabilitation, Urology, and Continuing Medical Education in the University of Minnesota Health Sciences Center, Vocational Technical Schools and other educational institutions, as well as by nursing associations and nursing homes, and commercial establishments devoted to training nursing assistants and other health care personnel.

Ellen Newman, M.T. (A.S.C.P.), M.S., was then and continues to be the director of the educational program in addition to her duties as associate scientist and bacteriologist in the Renal Function Laboratory of the Department of Physical Medicine and Rehabilitation. Working with her was Mary Price, M.D., Director of the Renal Function Laboratory and Associate Professor of Physical Medicine and Rehabilitation. Doctor Price is currently analyzing the data obtained during the comprehensive program of spinal cord injury follow-up. This material will be included in a future publication.

They were joined in 1974 by Jean Magney, M.S., former occupational therapist and at the time scientific illustrator but now Instructor in Anatomy. At first, Mrs. Magney planned slides, illustrations, and other visual aids for the project but later contributed lectures.

In 1976 the three published a manual, *Urinary Tract Care,* which has been widely distributed throughout the world. Although first intended as a "how to" book for patients, the manual has been used by many health professionals, some of whom have asked for a book which could be used as a quick reference for instruction in urinary tract care but which would also deal with causation of urinary tract dysfunction, the complications arising from poor function and its improper care, and the outcomes of various types of treatment. This volume is the result.

Mrs. Magney writes about the anatomy and pathology of the urinary tract and has illustrated the book. Doctor Price discusses the effects of pathology upon function, complications which may arise, and pharmacological management. Mrs. Newman deals with the most frequently used methods of urinary tract drainage and provides detailed instructions and rationale for each method. She also presents the principles of infection control and indicates the role of each discipline in the management of urinary tract care.

Because the authors hope that this book will prove useful to workers with widely varying backgrounds and experience, a glossary has been included. We realize that the book may be used as a ready reference by health care workers, and so an index has been included to direct the reader to specific areas of interest. Considerable repetition will be encountered from chapter to chapter. This has been deliberate to make each chapter self-contained, minimizing as much as possible the need to constantly refer to other sections. However, where the amount of material is lengthy, the reader will be referred to specific sections of other chapters.

Although we have made an effort to avoid the use of confusing abbreviations, we have followed many technical terms with abbreviations in common use, so that an uninitiated reader might more easily understand such references when encountered in medical speech and literature (e.g. cystometrogram) (CMG).

The use of proprietary names of drugs, supplies, or apparatus should not be construed to be a recommendation of those products over any others.

We hope that this volume will prove to be a valuable addition to the libraries of health care institutions, of workers involved in the long-term treatment of neurologically impaired individuals, and of the disabled individual. We have written it with the thought in mind that if everyone involved, from physician and nurse or other health professional, to the patient, thoroughly understands the principles underlying good urinary tract maintenance, a successful outcome will be realized. With such understanding, a disabled urinary tract no longer need be a threat to life.

E.N.
M.P.
J.M.

ACKNOWLEDGMENTS

We wish to acknowledge the contribution of the many individuals who read parts of this manuscript, offered helpful suggestions and/or assisted in its preparation. In alphabetical order, they include:

Eleanor Anderson, R.N., M.P.H.
Marilyn Barton
Saul Boyarsky, M.D.
Stanley Erlandsen, Ph.D.
Elvin E. Fraley, M.D.
Dolly Hewitt, R.N.
Christine Howard, J.D.
Frederic J. Kottke, M.D., Ph.D.
Patricia Lentsch, M.P.H., R.N.
Ursula Lommen, L.P.N.
Garland Meadows, M.Ed.
Lynn Newman
Jonathan Parsons, Ph.D.
Donna Pauley, R.P.T.
Thomas Thompson, M.S.
Mary Tuinenga, O.T.R.
Maj-Siri Ulmen
Marla Salmon, Sc.D., R.N., F.A.A.N.
Barbara Wiegand, R.P.T.

We are grateful to our husbands, Louis L. Bensman, M.D., Robert G. Magney, Raymond P. Newman, M.S.W., A.C.S.W., and to our families for their support and encouragement.

CONTENTS

CARE OF THE
DISABLED URINARY TRACT

Chapter I

ANATOMY AND PATHOLOGY
OF THE URINARY SYSTEM

ANATOMY OF THE KIDNEY AND URINARY TRACT

Kidney

Cut the kidney and note well its filtration, and where the blood separates from the urine, and where originates the gravel and the stone, and why . . . " (Leonardo da Vinci). Knowing "why" is the key to the successful rehabilitation of individuals with chronic urinary tract dysfunction. An understanding of the structure and function of the organs involved in urine formation and excretion is central to an intelligent response to the problems confronting these people on a day-to-day basis. Much of this book will deal with the bladder, because care of this organ is important in preserving the function of the kidneys which are essential to life.

Briefly, the function of the urinary tract is to remove certain waste products of metabolism from the body and to maintain the various constituents of the blood plasma, and its pH, at relatively constant levels. Approximately one-fifth of the body's total blood supply passes through the paired kidneys every minute, resulting in 170 liters of filtrate per day. Only 1.5 liters are normally excreted as urine. In a part of the kidney called the nephron, water and substances (such as sugars, salts, and small proteins) in simple solution are passed through a filtration barrier into a tubular system. Because some of the filtered substances are useful, they are reabsorbed through the walls of the tubule and conserved. Waste products, excess water, and some salts remain in the tubular system. Toxins and foreign substances, such as drugs, are transferred into it, and all are concentrated into urine. The ureters are muscular tubes which convey the urine from kidneys to the bladder, a hollow, expansile organ which is capable of accumulating a quantity of urine before emptying it into the urethra for elimination. Reflex urination occurs in infants, but in the normal adult the mature nervous system allows emptying at convenient intervals.

Macroanatomy

The kidneys lie on either side of the vertebral column between vertebral levels T12 and L2 (Plate I-1). These bean-shaped organs are approximately 10 cm long by 5 cm wide and are about 2.5 cm thick. A tough connective tissue capsule covers each organ, and it lies in a bed of fat, surrounded in turn by renal fascia, all of which offer protection. The drainage tube of the kidney, the ureter, together with renal blood and lymphatic vessels and a fine plexus of nerves reach the organ through a medially oriented concave fissure called the hilum. Within is the renal sinus which contains a funnel-shaped sac called the renal pelvis, and extensions of the pelvis called calyces (cups). These cups collect the urine which is then drained through the renal pelvis into the ureter.

Microanatomy

If one "cuts the kidney," it is seen to be subdivided into areas known as cortex and medulla (Plate I-2). The renal medulla is made up of conical masses of tissue known as pyramids. These structures are oriented with bases toward the capsule, and apices toward the renal pelvis. The apex is known as the papilla and is perforated by the collecting ducts, through which urine flows into the cup-like calyx. The base of each pyramid is covered with cortical tissue, which also extends down between the pyramids as the renal columns of Bertin.

Within the cortex and medulla lie the nephrons, the microscopic functional units of the kidney (Plate I-3). Nephrons are made up of renal corpuscles and tubules. The renal corpuscle, which lies in the cortex, consists of a tuft of looped capillaries, the glomerulus (Fig. I-1), which has pushed into the blind end of the tubule as a fist might push into a partially inflated balloon. As a result, a layer of tubular epithelium closely invests the glomerulus and then loosely folds back upon itself to form Bowman's capsule. The space between the epithelium which adheres to the glomerulus (visceral epithelium) and that of the outer capsule wall (parietal epithelium) is called Bowman's (urinary) space. This space receives the filtrate and drains into the tubule of the nephron (Plate I-4 and Fig. I-2).

The renal corpuscle has a vascular pole where the afferent arteriole, supplying the glomerular capillaries, enters. The capillaries receive blood from the afferent arteriole and drain into the efferent arteriole. This smaller vessel leaves the corpuscle at the vascular pole close to where the afferent vessel enters, and then breaks up into a second (peritubular) capillary bed. Opposite the vascular pole is the urinary pole, where Bowman's capsule narrows to become the proximal convoluted tubule (PCT).

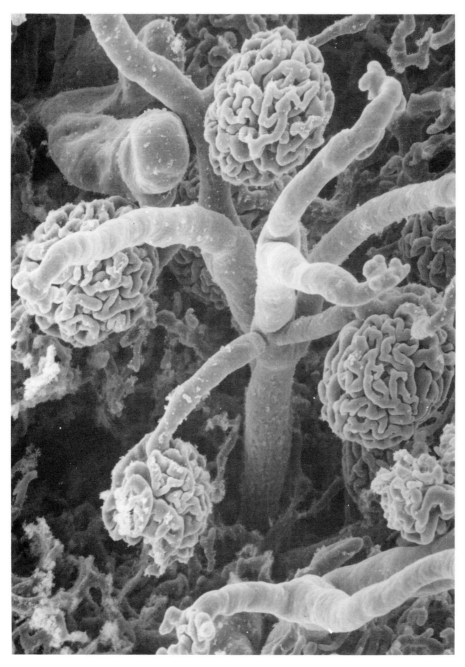

Figure I-1. A vascular cast of renal glomeruli and afferent arterioles as seen by scanning electron microscopy (SEM). Courtesy of Doctor Stanley L. Erlandsen, Department of Anatomy, University of Minnesota Medical School, Minneapolis, MN.

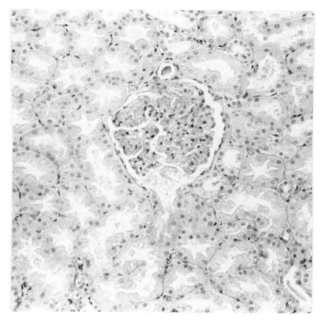

Figure I-2. Renal corpuscle and cortical labyrinth visualized by light microscopy (LM) (hematoxylin and eosin stain).

The proximal convoluted tubule pursues a tortuous course through the cortex, creating what is known as the cortical labyrinth (Plate I-5). The proximal tubule then straightens and enters the medulla, where it narrows to become the descending limb of the loop of Henle. Penetration of the medulla is variable. Cortical nephrons (with corpuscles near the capsule) have short loops, while juxtamedullary nephrons (with corpuscles near the corticomedullary junction) deeply penetrate the pyramid. After making a hairpin bend, the ascending limb of the loop of Henle thickens, re-enters the cortex, passes near the corpuscle of origin, and becomes the distal convoluted tubule (DCT). After a winding course through the cortex, the distal convoluted tubule empties into the collecting duct which descends on a straight course through cortex and medulla, and opens, as previously described, through the renal papilla into a calyx.

Blood Supply

The blood supply of the kidney is essential to its function. A direct branch of the aorta, called the renal artery, serves each kidney (see Plate I-2). As this vessel approaches the hilum, it divides into five segmental arteries which provide for discrete areas of the organ. These in turn branch into interlobar arteries which course toward the capsule in the renal columns which lie between the medullary pyramids (see Plate I-5). At the corticomedullary junction the interlobar arteries give off branches called arcuate arteries which ramify over the base of the pyramid and divide in turn into interlobular arteries. These vessels again course toward the capsule and supply the glomeruli with afferent arterioles. The interlobular arteries terminate as capillaries in the capsule.

Juxtaglomerular Apparatus

The afferent arteriole is a large thick-walled vessel with specialized secretory muscle cells in its wall. These special cells of the afferent arteriole, a dense cluster of epithelial cells within the wall of the distal tubule (macula densa), and supporting cells comprise the juxtaglomerular apparatus which lies next to the glomerulus (Fig. I-3). Under conditions of low blood pressure and/or reduced osmolarity, the secretory muscle fibers release a proteolytic enzyme, called renin, into the blood. Renin converts a plasma protein, angiotensinogen, to angiotensin I, which is in turn converted to angiotensin II, presumably by the action of a converting enzyme in the lung. Angiotensin II causes systemic arteriolar constriction, thereby raising blood pressure. It also stimulates the secretion of aldosterone by the adrenal cortex. Aldosterone raises blood pressure by causing conservation of salt (and, secondarily, water) by the distal tubule.

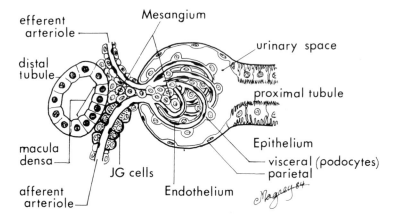

Figure I-3. Juxtaglomerular apparatus in relationship to renal corpuscle.

Filtration Barrier

As previously described, the afferent arteriole branches into a tuft of capillaries, called the glomerulus. The cells of the capillary walls, the cells of the tubular epithelium which closely envelopes the capillaries, and their fused basement membranes make up the filtration barrier (Figs. I-4 and I-5). The endothelial cells which form the capillary wall are pierced by small openings called fenestrae which permit passage of some substances but which retain the larger constituents of the blood, such as large plasma proteins and blood cells, within the vessel. The principle barriers to filtration are the fused basement membranes which consist of a network of interlacing fibrils acting as a fine sieve, and associated negatively charged molecules that constitute a charge barrier.[1-5] Finally, the cells of the tubule (visceral epithelium) which have been modified to provide support to the capillary loops exhibit interlocking cytoplasmic processes separated by small spaces called filtration slits. These are usually bridged by diaphragms and offer the last barrier to filtration. A substance which negotiates this combination of obstacles arrives in Bowman's space and drains from there into the tubular part of the nephron at the urinary pole.

By virtue of its thick muscular walls, the afferent arteriole sends blood into the glomerulus at relatively high hydrostatic pressure. The movement of substances from the capillary through the filtration barrier and into Bowman's space is promoted by the relatively lower resistance to flow offered by Bowman's space. The volume of fluid passing through the filtration barrier per minute is called the glomerular filtration rate (GFR).

Microcirculation

Capillaries of the glomerulus reunite to form the efferent arteriole which emerges from the vascular pole of the renal corpuscle and then breaks up into a second bed of capillaries (Plate I-5). If the renal corpuscle is located peripherally in the cortex near the capsule (cortical nephron), the capillaries which derive from the efferent arteriole provide for the cortically situated tubules and are called peritubular capillaries. If the renal corpuscle lies near the medulla (juxtamedullary nephron), the capillaries arising from the efferent arteriole course into the medulla in parallel with the loops of Henle, and are called vasa recta (straight vessels). Both groups of vessels are important to tubular reabsorption and secretion.

The secondary capillary beds reunite, forming venules which drain into interlobular or arcuate veins, depending on their location. Subsequent drainage is by way of interlobar, segmental, and renal veins into the inferior vena cava.

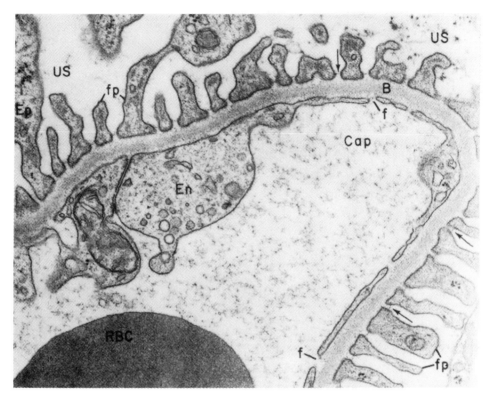

Figure I-4. Transmission electron micrograph (TEM) of filtration barrier, renal corpuscle: RBC, red blood cell; En, endothelial cell; Cap, capillary; B, basement membrane; f, fenestration; fp, foot processes of podocyte; Ep, epithelial cell (podocyte); US, urinary space. Courtesy of Doctor Marilyn Gist Farquhar. Reprinted with permission from *Kidney International* 8:197–211, 1975.

Lymphatics

Lymphatic capillaries are seen in relationship to the blood vessels of the kidney beginning at the level of the interlobular arteries. Anastomotic connections exist between these tiny vessels and the rich lymphatic supply of the kidney capsule and perirenal tissues. Lymphatic drainage is toward the hilum of the kidney, with the smaller vessels combining in the renal sinus to form large channels which pass through aortic nodes and into the thoracic duct.

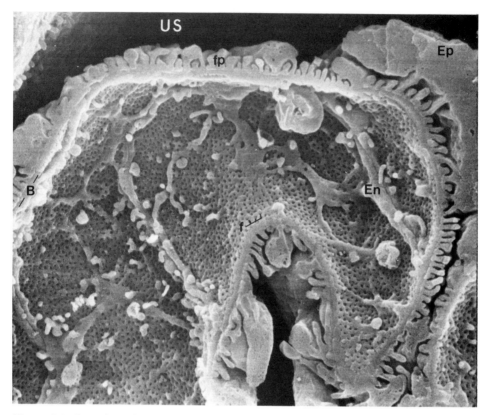

Figure I-5. Scanning electron micrograph (SEM) of filtration barrier showing the same structures as seen in Figure I-4. The glomerular capillary loop has been cut in longitudinal section so that the luminal surface of the endothelium is exposed. Numerous fenestrae are seen in the endothelium: En, ridge of cytoplasm of endothelial cell; B, basement membrane; f, fenestrae; fp, foot processes (of podocyte); Ep, epithelial cell (podocyte); US, urinary space. Courtesy of Doctor Tsuneo Fujita. Reprinted with permission from Fujita, Tanaka, and Tokunaga, (Eds.): *SEM Atlas of Cells and Tissues.* Tokyo, Igaku Shoin Ltd., 1981.

Tubular Function

Of the 170 liters of glomerular filtrate produced daily, about 85 percent is reabsorbed by the proximal convoluted tubule and includes substances useful to the body, such as water, glucose, amino acids, sodium, and potassium (Table I-I). These pass into the intercellular compartment (interstitium) and from there diffuse into the peritubular capillaries to be recycled. Drugs and other foreign matter present in body fluids move from the capillaries through the interstitium and are transferred by the cells of the proximal convoluted tubule into the lumen of the tubule. This is called tubular excretion. Waste products of metabolism remain in the tubule to be concentrated into urine.

TABLE I-I
TUBULAR FUNCTION

Tubule	Reabsorption	H_2O/da	Secretion	Excretion
PCT: (Reabsorption of useful substances)	Salt (70%) Water Amino Acids Glucose Proteins Bicarbonate Urea	120 L	Organic acids and bases	Metabolic wastes and foreign materials
Loop: (Manufactures hypertonic medullary interstitium)	Salt Water	10 L		
D.T. (Regulates salt and acid base balance)	Salt Water Bicarbonate	20 L	Hydrogen Ammonium Potassium	
C.D. Cortex Medulla (concentrates urine)	Water Water	15 L 8 L		

Concentrated urine occurs only in animals whose kidneys possess loops of Henle. The mechanisms responsible are called countercurrent multiplier and countercurrent exchange and involve the loop of Henle, the distal convoluted tubule and the collecting duct. The word "countercurrent" describes the movement of fluid down into the medulla, around the bend, and up in the opposite ("counter") direction and out of the medulla. This occurs both in the loops of Henle and the vasa rectae.

The cells of the ascending limb of the loop of Henle are impermeable to water but actively pump salt out of the tubule into the medullary interstitium, which becomes hypertonic with respect to blood plasma. As the descending limb is freely permeable to both water and solutes, water is drawn from the tubule by the hypertonic interstitium, causing the remaining tubular fluid to become increasingly concentrated. As salt is pumped out of the nearby ascending limb, it diffuses into the descending limb, turns the bend into the ascending limb, and is again pumped out of the tubule. This is the countercurrent multiplier, responsible for the osmotic gradient which concentrates the fluid in the descending limb and, as we shall see, in the collecting duct.

As the fluid which has been partially concentrated in the descending limb moves up the ascending limb, salt is removed by the sodium pump, so that the fluid reaching the cortex is hypotonic with respect to plasma. The filtrate now enters the distal convoluted tubule. Here, sodium is reabsorbed under the influence of aldosterone, controlling salt and water balance in the body. The cells of the distal convoluted tubule also secrete hydrogen ions and ammonium ions into the filtrate, and reabsorb bicarbonate to maintain the acid-base balance of the blood and to acidify the urine.

Final concentration of urine takes place in the collecting duct under the influence of antidiuretic hormone (ADH). This hormone is synthesized by cells of the hypothalamus and released as needed by the posterior pituitary gland. Insufficient water intake or excessive sweating produces blood which is low in water content. This is sensed by osmoreceptors in the hypothalamus and causes the release of antidiuretic hormone. Carried by the blood to the kidney, antidiuretic hormone acts upon the walls of the collecting duct to make it permeable to water. Because the collecting duct descends through the medulla to open at the papilla, it is exposed along its length to the increasingly hypertonic medullary environment. As a consequence, water is lost from the urine (which becomes increasingly concentrated) and conserved by the body. In the absence of antidiuretic hormone, the walls of the collecting duct are impermeable to water and the urine is overabundant and hypotonic.

A countercurrent exchange mechanism is formed by the vasa rectae which run in parallel with the loops of Henle. Salt enters the vessels as they descend into the medulla, but is lost by diffusion as they ascend, and water is exchanged, as well. This countercurrent blood flow permits vascular supply to the medulla without disruption of the hypertonic medullary environment.

Innervation

The kidneys are innervated by both divisions of the autonomic nervous system. The middle and inferior splanchnic nerves (T10,11,12) and the first lumbar splanchnic nerves (L1,2) supply preganglionic sympathetic fibers to celiac, aorticorenal, and renal perivascular plexuses. Postganglionic fibers travel with the blood vessels into the kidney. The vagus and pelvic splanchnic nerves provide parasympathetic innervation. There is no good evidence for any important nervous function in the kidney other than vasomotor activity and the conduction of pain, although some workers believe that these nerves may provide a feedback mechanism through baroreceptors in the carotid sinus and aortic arch to control renal perfusion pressure.

Excretory Passages

The excretory passages of the urinary tract share a histologically similar structure, although an increase in size and a thickening of the wall is apparent distally. All are lined with transitional epithelium which is unique to the urinary tract. The epithelium also increases in thickness from 2–3 cells in the calyces and 4–5 in the ureter to 6–8 cells in the contracted bladder.

Connective tissue binds the epithelium to the smooth muscle coat. In the ureter, the smooth muscle bundles are arranged in inner longitudinal and outer circular layers. This arrangement is partially lost in the bladder, where bundles are interwoven and the walls very thick. There is also increased connective tissue between the muscle bundles of the bladder. In both organs, an adventitial layer of connective tissue covers the muscularis (muscle layer). However, a serosa (of peritoneum) supplants the adventitia on the anterior surface of the ureters and the superior surface of the bladder.

The epithelium of the relaxed bladder exhibits luminal "dome" or "umbrella" cells (Fig. I-6). These cells bulge into the lumen and have interdigitating lateral borders joined to adjacent cells by tight junctions which allow the cell to stretch and flatten when the bladder fills while maintaining a barrier between the hypertonic, toxic urine and the bladder tissue.

By transmission electron microscopy, the luminal membranes of these cells appear thickened and folded with regions of membrane in circular or polygonal plaques joined by membrane of normal thickness at the folds.[6] The cytoplasm of luminal cells contains numerous discoid vesicles with structural similarities to the plaques of the luminal membrane (Fig. I-7). These vesicles may unite to form chains of vesicles which fuse with the luminal membrane. In this manner, additional surface membrane may be added to the expanding bladder. Upon bladder contraction, plaques are internalized and stored as discoid vesicles within the cytoplasm. This also provides a mechanism for adding newly synthesized membrane to the cell or removing old membrane from an epithelium which is constantly exposed to toxic urine (Fig. I-8).[6]

Ureters

The renal pelvis emerges from the hilum of the kidney and narrows to become the ureter. A ureter drains each kidney, conveying the urine to the bladder. Although they course from the kidneys high in the abdomen to the bladder deep in the pelvis, gravity is not the principle force moving urine along these tubes. Two layers of smooth muscle within the walls of the

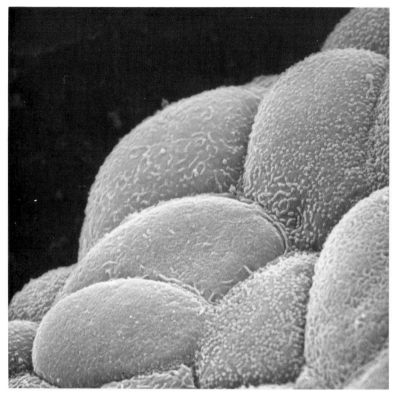

Figure I-6. Scanning electron micrograph of transitional epithelium. The epithelial cells are seen to bulge into the lumen and are called dome cells. They flatten when the wall of the organ is stretched.

ureters are arranged to perform this function. Contraction of the inner, longitudinally oriented layer pulls the tube over a quantity (bolus) of urine, much as a sock is pulled on over the foot. Subsequently, the outer, circular layer squeezes in on the bolus, "milking" it along the ureter toward the bladder. This action, called peristalsis, makes it possible for urine to be moved in the correct direction, regardless of the position of the body. It also normally prevents regurgitation of urine from bladder toward the kidney (reflux), which might introduce bacteria from the bladder into the kidney. The muscular contractions of the ureter are modulated by the autonomic nervous system, but peristalsis appears to be intrinsic, for if the ureters are denervated, it persists. Alpha and beta adrenoreceptors have both been recognized in the ureteral muscle; however, it is possible that myogenic contractions may be modulated by circulating catecholamines, as myoneural synapses have not been seen.[7] The ureters increase in size from kidney to bladder. Obstruction by stones (calculi) occurs most often in parts of the

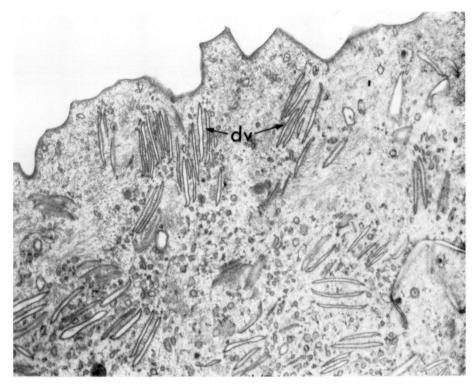

Figure I-7. Transmission electron micrograph of transitional epithelial cells. Excess plasma-lemma (cell membrane) is stored within the cell's cytoplasm as discoid vesicles (dv) which are reinserted into the surface membrane as the bladder fills. Courtesy of Doctor Keith R. Porter. Reprinted with permission from *Protoplasma* 63:262, 1967.

tube which are normally somewhat constricted (Fig. I-9). Such sites are the ureteropelvic junction (where renal pelvis narrows to become the ureter), the place where the ureter crosses the iliac vessels, and the intramural course of the ureter.

A ureter descends from the kidney along the length of the psoas muscle, crossing the iliac vessels as it passes into the pelvis just lateral to the sacroiliac joint (Plate I-1). Its course is entirely extraperitoneal. In the female, the ureter approaches the posterior of the bladder, through the broad ligament of the uterus, and passes near the uterine cervix, where it is crossed superiorly by the uterine vessels. After running close to the lateral fornix of the vagina, it enters the posterosuperior angle of the bladder. In the male, the ureter passes through the sacrogenital fold toward the postero-superior angle of the bladder, which it joins just lateral and inferior to the ductus deferens.

In both male and female, the course of the ureter through the bladder

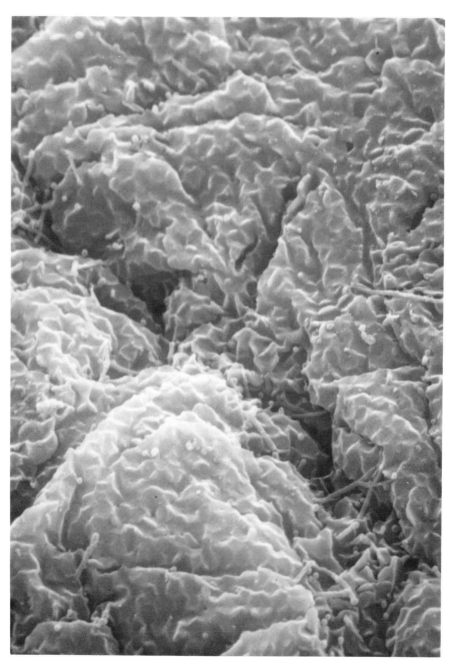

Figure 1-8. High magnification scanning electron micrograph of bladder surface revealing discoidal vesicle membrane in plasmalemma of dome cells. Courtesy of Doctor Stanley L. Erlandsen, Department of Anatomy, University of Minnesota Medical School, Minneapolis, MN.

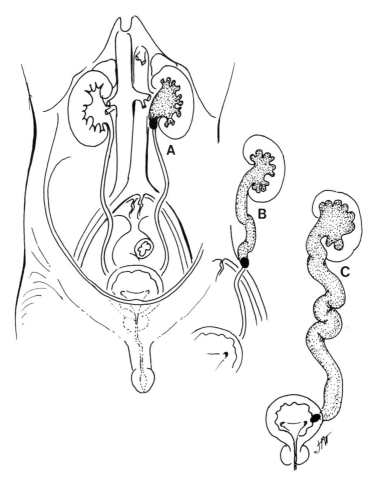

Figure I-9. Sites within the urinary tract where stones often cause obstruction. A. Ureteropelvic junction. B. Ureter as it crosses iliac vessels at pelvic brim. C. Intramural course of ureter through bladder wall.

wall is from posterosuperior to anteromedial. This diagonal intramural course, and a valve-like fold of the mucous membrane lining the bladder have been thought to prevent the reflux of urine. However, recent studies involving the microdissection of the ureterovesical junction suggest a more complex arrangement. The inner longitudinal muscle layer of the ureter penetrates the bladder wall and blends with its innermost muscle. As peristaltic waves of contraction sweep down the ureter, this inner muscle layer opens the intramural segment of the ureteral lumen, allowing urine to pass into the bladder. Muscle fibers of both ureteral and vesical (bladder) origin wrap in a spiral fashion around the intramural ureter, and a superficial spiral sheath of outermost bladder muscle ascends the ureter for a few centimeters. Internally, the innermost bladder muscle sends fibers across and around the outlet of the ureter. As bladder muscle contracts to empty the organ, sheath fibers of bladder origin also contract, compressing the intramural segments of the ureters and preventing reflux of urine.[8,9]

Bladder (Vesical)

The bladder is a hollow muscular organ that lies in the true pelvis posterior to the pubic bones (Plate I-6). It has a domed, posterosuperior portion called the fundus, which narrows anteriorly to the apex. The body of the bladder lies posteroinferiorly and contains in its posterior wall the two ureteral orifices. The organ narrows inferiorly to the neck, or bladder outlet, which contains the urethral orifice. The area demarcated by these three openings constitutes the trigone.

Superiorly, the bladder is covered by a reflection of peritoneum from the anterior abdominal wall which is carried posteriorly to the rectum. The bladder is attached to the lateral pelvic walls by adventitia (connective tissue) and a variety of fibrous strands called "true ligaments."

In the male, the prostate gland, immediately below the bladder neck, is bound to it by strong fibrous attachments. The posterior bladder wall is in close relationship to the paired seminal vesicles and the ampullae of the deferent ducts, and with them is separated from the rectum by the retrovesical fascia of Denonvilliers. Sacrogenital folds of peritoneum sweep posteriorly and enfold the terminal ureters.

In the female, the bladder is closely apposed posteriorly to the vagina, with which it shares the vesicovaginal septum (Plate I-7). The uterus normally lies behind and above the fundus of the bladder. Peritoneum covers bladder and uterus, and the sacrogenital folds in the female sweep from the uterus to the rectum and contain the terminal portion of the ureters. These peritoneal folds are called "false ligaments."

Innervation

The bladder and lower ureters are supplied by sympathetic fibers from spinal cord segments T12, L1 and L2 which descend in the hypogastric plexus (Plate I-8). Postganglionic neurons of this division may be found in the inferior mesenteric ganglia or in ganglia associated with the hypogastric or vesical plexuses. The sacral outflow (S2,3,4) supplies parasympathetic fibers by way of the pelvic nerves to bladder and lower ureters where postganglionic neurons lie in clusters within the walls of the organs (Fig. I-10). Studies involving the micturition reflex[8,10,11] indicate triple innervation of the internal sphincter (bladder outlet) and external sphincter, with both sympathetic and parasympathetic ganglia seen intramurally, as well as interganglionic connections between them. Somatic innervation of the external sphincter is through the pudendal nerves from S2, 3 and 4 (Plate I-8).

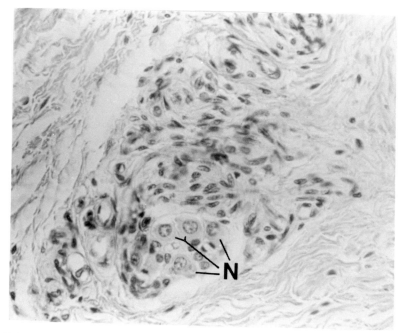

Figure I-10. Light micrograph of postganglionic neurons in connective tissue septa of bladder wall (hematoxylin and eosin stain).

Parasympathetic neurons release the neurotransmitter acetylcholine, and their receptor sites are called cholinergic. The effect of this neurotransmitter is to cause the detrusor muscle to contract and the bladder to empty.

Sympathetic nerves reaching the bladder, ureters and urethra release the neurotransmitter noradrenalin which crosses the synapse and binds to the muscle cell membrane at receptor sites where it induces physiological changes in the muscle cell. Alpha-adrenergic receptors mediate contraction of smooth muscle, while beta-adrenergic receptors mediate smooth muscle relaxation.[7, 12]

Alpha- and beta-adrenergic receptor populations are not uniformly distributed in the lower urinary tract (Fig. I-11). Alpha receptors are found principally in the base of the bladder, near the urethral orifice, in the trigone and proximal urethra.[13–15] In these positions they mediate contraction (closure) of the internal sphincter and urethral muscle, leading to continence. Beta receptors, on the other hand, are found primarily in the detrusor muscle of the body and fundus of the bladder, where they act to relax the muscle wall, allowing the organ to fill and increasing bladder volume capacity. Some investigators have seen beta receptors in the bladder base and neck and think that beta-adrenergic receptor function opens the internal sphincter.[13] The effect of noradrenalin may be dose dependent, with large doses causing contraction (alpha receptors) and low doses causing relaxation (beta receptors).

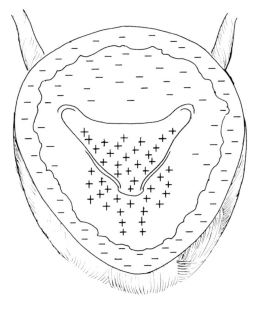

+ :   α adrenergic receptors

− :   β adrenergic receptors

Figure I-11. Adrenergic receptor populations in the bladder.

In addition, it appears that ganglion cells of the pelvic plexus respond to both parasympathetic and sympathetic preganglionic input. This would suggest that the parasympathetic impulses which cause detrusor contraction may secondarily cause activation at the bladder outlet of beta-adrenergic receptors, resulting in relaxation of the internal sphincter.[13]

Drugs may be used to mimic the effect of neurotransmitters and are called sympathomimetic drugs when they mimic noradrenalin. The contractile activity of the bladder can be affected by the choice of therapeutic drugs, which if they bind to alpha-adrenergic receptors will cause contraction or if they bind to beta-adrenergic receptors will cause relaxation. Drugs may also be used to block the effects of contraction or relaxation by blockading the receptors.[12, 16]

The bladder rests upon a sling of striated muscle called the pelvic diaphragm (Plates I-6 and I-7). Because part of this striated (voluntary) muscle surrounds the urethra, its tonic contraction results in closure of that tubular organ. This is also called the urogenital diaphragm, or external sphincter, and is innervated by the somatic nervous system through fibers of the pudendal nerve from spinal cord segments S2, 3, and 4. The neurotransmitter at the neuromuscular junction is acetylcholine. Parasympathetic and sympathetic fibers have also been identified in the external sphincter, and sympathetic fibers are seen to run between the striated muscle cells in close approximation to their surfaces. Smooth muscle cells are also in evidence. Some investigators believe that this sphincter may be primarily under the influence of the alpha-adrenergic innervation and that disturbances are probably autonomic.[11,17]

The act of micturition is therefore the result of coordination of nervous impulses arising from several divisions of the nervous system. This complex innervation may lead to disturbances of micturition if parts of the nerve supply are affected by trauma or disease (neurogenic bladder). On the other hand, drugs may be used therapeutically to modify the contractile activities of bladder and urethra.

As the bladder fills (Fig. I-12), pressure and stretch receptors in its wall respond to changing volume and pressure and send impulses over sensory fibers of the pelvic nerves to S2, 3, and 4 levels of the spinal cord. A reflex arc is established with motor neurons of the parasympathetic division which transmit to the detrusor muscle of the bladder causing it to rhythmically contract. The desire to urinate is recognized by transmission to cortical levels of the brain, and urination may be voluntarily delayed to an appropriate time and place by inhibition of detrusor contraction and conscious reinforcement of the external sphincter. When appropriate, the tonic contraction of the external sphincter is inhibited, detrusor contractions resume, and the bladder is emptied (Fig. I-13).

Visceral pain (pain arising in an organ such as the bladder or urethra) reaches the central nervous system by way of fibers which run (in reverse direction) with both the hypogastric plexus and the pelvic nerves (Plate I-8). Precise localization of visceral pain is impossible, due to lack of touch receptors in deep structures such as the internal organs. This results in the referral of pain from deep structures to the body wall and can be explained only by the fact that skin and deep organs share segmental innervation (Fig. I-14). Sensation from the pelvic diaphragm travels in afferent fibers of the pudendal nerves.

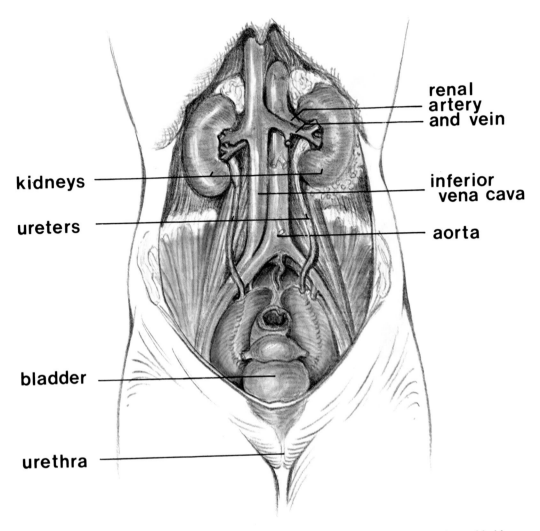

renal
artery
and vein

kidneys

inferior
vena cava

ureters

aorta

bladder

urethra

Plate I-1. The urinary system within the abdominopelvic cavity. Kidneys, ureters, urinary bladder and urethra are shown in the female.

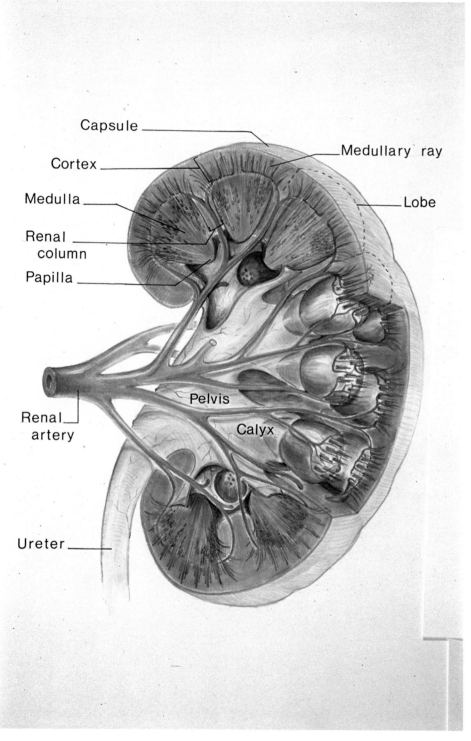

Plate I-2. Hemisected kidney, renal pelvis, and blood supply.

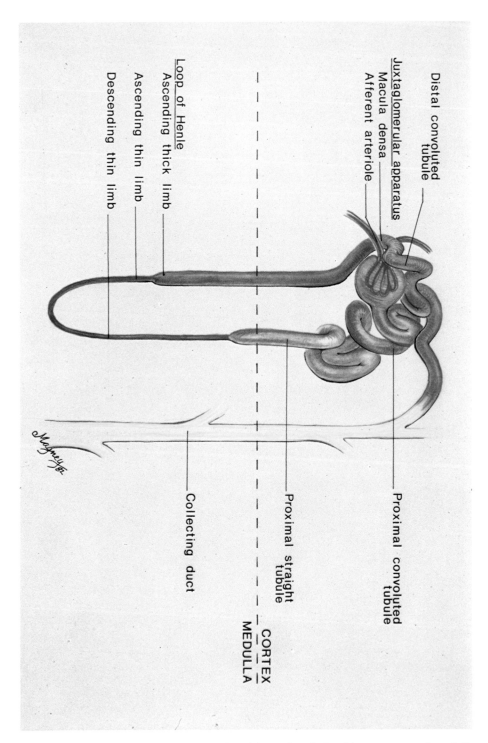

Plate I-3. Nephron, the functional unit of the kidney, in relationship to cortex and medulla.

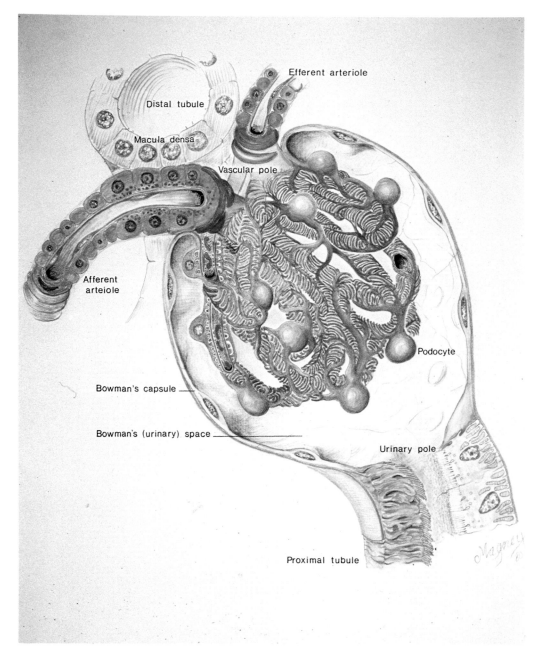

Plate I-4. Renal corpuscle, made up of glomerulus and Bowman's capsule.

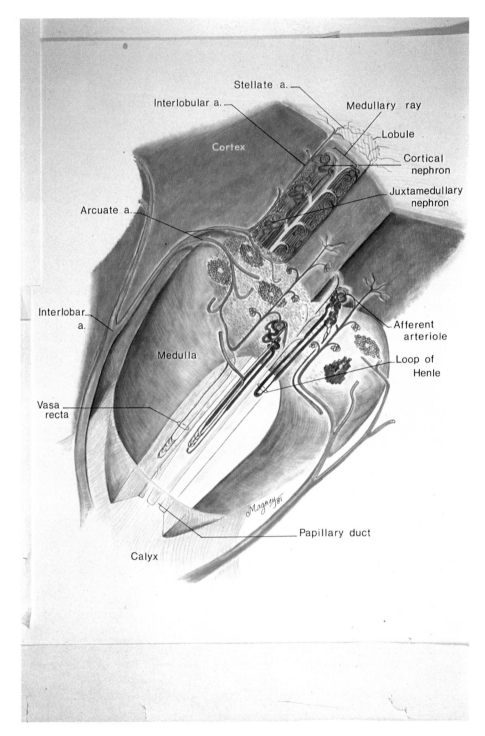

Plate I-5. Details of renal cortex and medulla showing disposition of nephrons and blood vessels.

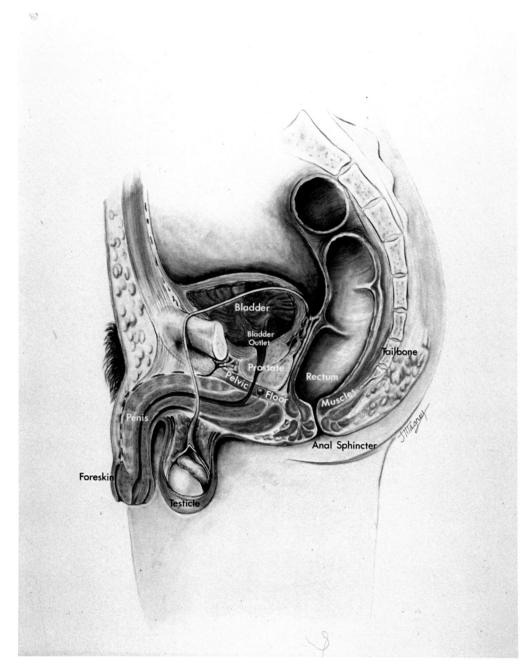

Plate I-6. Lateral view of the pelvic organs of the male.

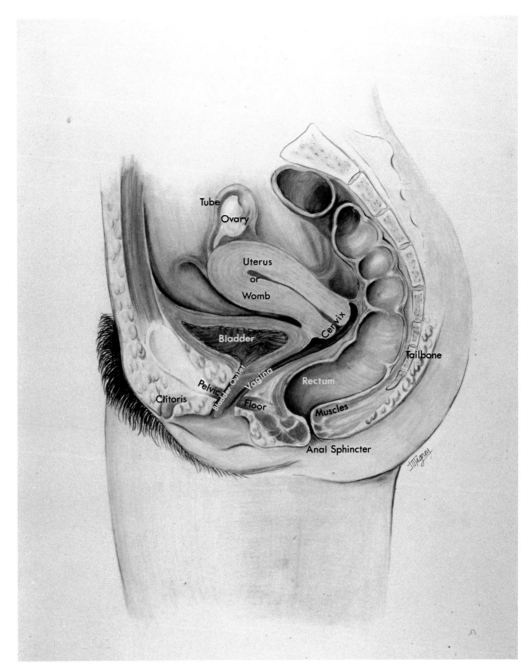

Labels in image: Tube, Ovary, Uterus or Womb, Cervix, Bladder, Tailbone, Pelvic Floor, Bladder Outlet, Vagina, Rectum, Clitoris, Floor, Muscles, Anal Sphincter

Plate I-7. Lateral view of the pelvic organs of the female.

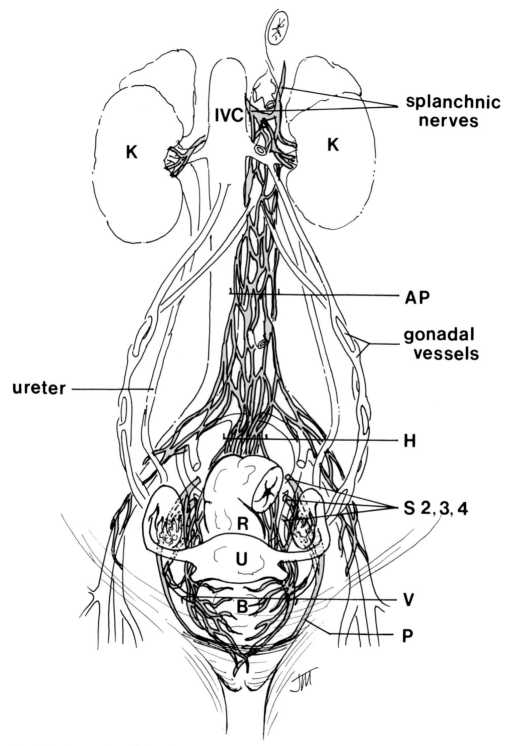

Plate I-8. Innervation of the urinary tract. AP, aortic plexus; H, hypogastric plexus; V, vesical plexus; P, pudendal nerve; K, kidneys; IVC, inferior vena cava; U, uterus; B, bladder; R, rectum.

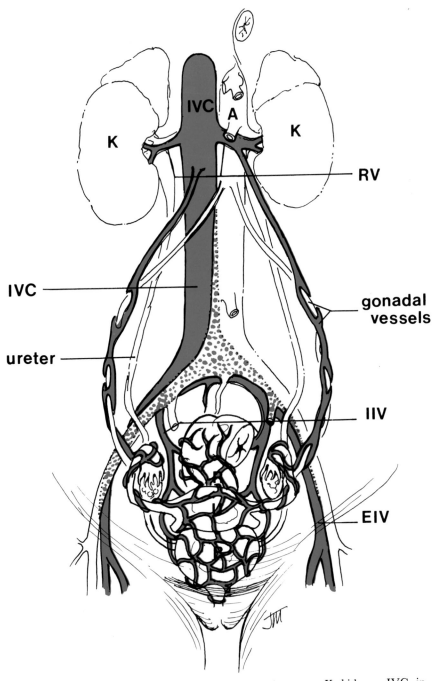

Plate I-9. Venous drainage of urinary tract and pelvic organs. K, kidneys; IVC, inferior vena cava; RV, renal veins; A, aorta; IIV, internal iliac veins.

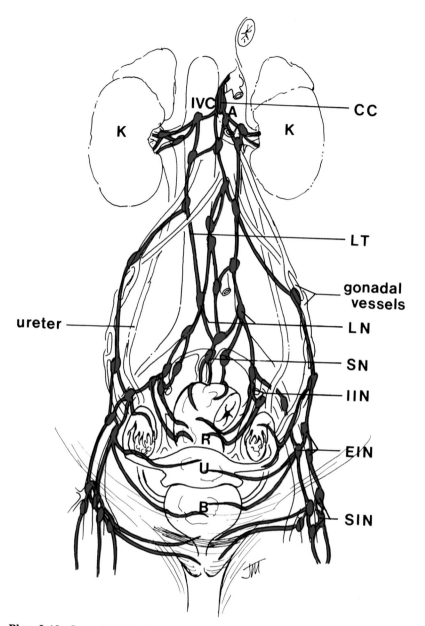

Plate I-10. Lymphatic drainage of urinary tract and pelvic organs. K, kidneys; U, uterus; B, bladder; IVC, inferior vena cava; A, aorta; R, rectum; SIN, superficial inguinal nodes; EIN, external iliac nodes; IIN, internal iliac nodes; SN, sacral nodes; LN, lumbar nodes; LT, lumbar trunks; CC, cysterna chyli.

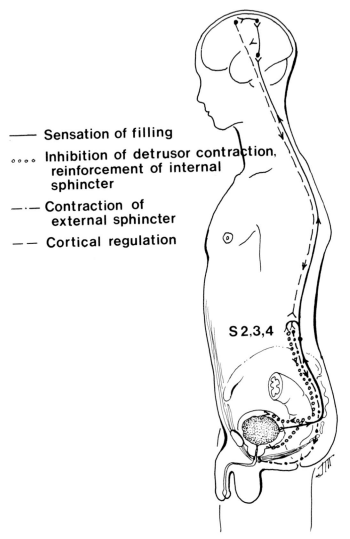

——— Sensation of filling

∘∘∘∘ Inhibition of detrusor contraction, reinforcement of internal sphincter

—·— Contraction of external sphincter

— — Cortical regulation

S 2,3,4

Figure I-12. Micturition reflex is inhibited by neurons in the brain which modulate reflex activity in spinal cord segments S2, 3, and 4.

Musculature

The inner longitudinal layer of ureteral smooth muscle continues into the bladder as the superficial muscle layer of the trigone and, further, into the proximal urethra as its internal longitudinal muscle (Fig. I-15A). The smooth muscle which makes up most of the bladder wall has a different embryonic derivation and is called detrusor muscle. In addition to body

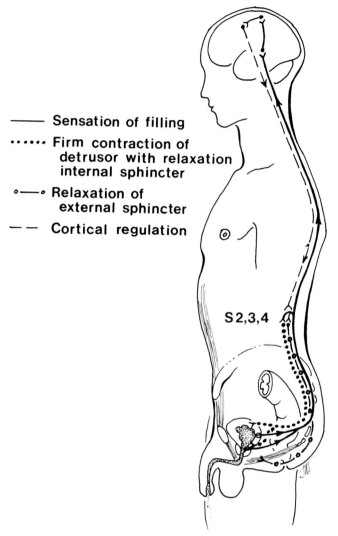

Sensation of filling

Firm contraction of detrusor with relaxation internal sphincter

Relaxation of external sphincter

Cortical regulation

S 2,3,4

Figure I-13. The bladder is emptied at the appropriate time and place as determined by cortical centers.

and fundus, the detrusor muscle also forms the deep trigone, Waldeyers sheath (which extends up and around the lower ureter), and the outer circular layer of urethral musculature. In the bladder, the detrusor is disposed roughly in three layers.[18]

An inner, longitudinal layer is very thin, with widely separated fibers and an interwoven arrangement, except at the bladder neck, where the fibers blend with the inner longitudinal layer of urethral muscle (Fig. I-15B).

A middle, circular, thick layer terminates at the bladder neck. It forms

Bladder - <u>Fundùs</u>
posterior view

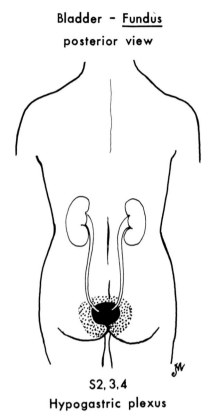

S2, 3, 4
Hypogastric plexus

Figure I-14. Referred pain. Noxious sensation from the bladder is perceived as pain surrounding the anus.

concentric rings about the bladder outlet (Fig. I-15C). The innermost rings are incomplete and blend posteriorly with the deep trigonal muscle, while the outer rings complete their loop behind the deep trigone. These rings of detrusor muscle circling the urethral orifice at the base of the bladder are sometimes called the "trigonal loop," or "fundus ring," and form what is known as the baseplate of the bladder. Under the primary influence of the alpha-adrenergic fibers of the sympathetic nervous system, the baseplate is in a tonic state of contraction which serves to close the internal sphincter.

An outer, longitudinal layer of detrusor muscle is located mainly anteriorly and posteriorly; the lateral walls are only thinly covered by this layer (Fig. I-15D). Anterior fibers of the outermost layer insert into an arc of fibrous connective tissue which lies just anterior to the proximal urethra. Posterior fibers are divided into a medial group which inserts into the trigone at the bladder neck (apex of the trigone) and into a lateral group whose fibers loop around the urethra from posterior to anterior, where they also blend with the anterior arc of connective tissue as well as with lateral posterior fibers from the opposite side. This loop forms the upper anterior wall of the urethra and is called the detrusor loop.

While the bladder is filling (Fig. I-16A), the baseplate is flat and the muscle in a state of tonic contraction, which, because of the disposition of the fibers of the trigonal loop, closes the internal sphincter. The rest of the detrusor, under the influence primarily of beta-adrenergic receptors, relaxes to allow filling.

At micturition (Fig. I-16B), parasympathetic impulses stimulate the outermost layer of detrusor to contract, and the medial posterior group, inserting at the apex of the trigone, pulls the posterior wall of the outlet back and upwards with an opening effect. The anterior group, assisted by the detrusor loop, pulls the anterior connective tissue arc upwards, breaking the flat baseplate and creating a funnel called the trigonal canal. Now the fundus ring contracts and, because of the change in shape of the bladder base, its contraction helps to maintain the trigonal canal. At the same time, contraction of the entire detrusor and inhibition of the external sphincter allow urination to take place.

Urethra

The male urethra, 18 to 20 cm long, is divided into prostatic, membranous, and penile parts (Plate I-6). The ejaculatory duct and prostatic glands open into the prostatic portion of the urethra which runs within the substance of that organ which lies immediately beneath the bladder. The membranous part of the urethra is surrounded by the striated muscle of the urogenital diaphragm (made up of pelvic outlet muscles), while the penile portion of the urethra passes longitudinally through the corpus spongiosum of the penis. The epithelium varies from transitional proximally to pseudostratified and stratified squamous distally, where it blends with the skin of the glans. The lamina propria is a loose, elastic connective tissue containing numerous bundles of smooth muscle longitudinally arranged. Outer circular muscle is also present.

The male external genitalia are the penis and the scrotum, a skin-covered fibromuscular sac which contains the testicles. The penis is made up of three erectile bodies, the corpora cavernosae, bound together by a connective tissue sheath. The corpus cavernosa urethra (also called corpus spongiosum) contains the urethra throughout its length and is enclosed by a more elastic connective tissue than are the two dorsal corpora cavernosae which are tightly bound by the tunica albuginea. The blood vessels supplying the vascular sinusoids of the cavernous bodies are called helicine arteries because they are coiled by the tonic contraction of the smooth muscle in their walls.

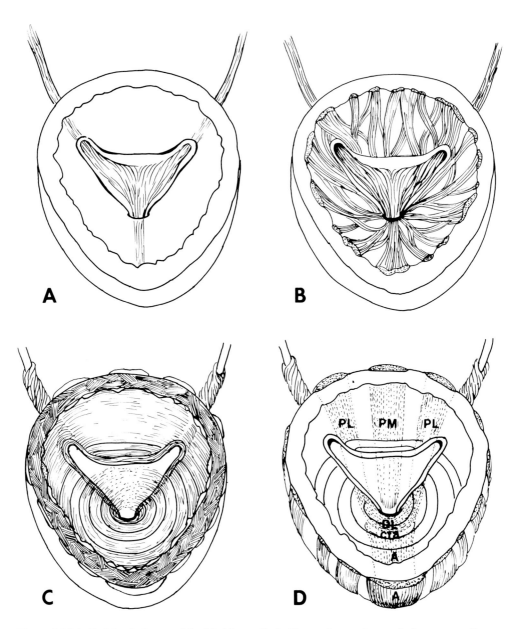

Figure I-15 A–D. Muscle layers of the bladder wall. A. Ureteral smooth muscle forms superficial trigone and continues into urethra. B. Inner, longitudinal layer of detrusor muscle. C. Middle, circular layer of detrusor forms the trigonal loop (fundus ring; baseplate) around bladder outlet and makes up bulk of bladder wall. D. A thin, outer longitudinal layer is condensed posteriorly and anteriorly into groups of fibers which control the bladder outlet (internal sphincter). PM, posteromedial group; PL, posterolateral group; A, anterior group; CTA, connective tissue arc; DL, detrusor loop.

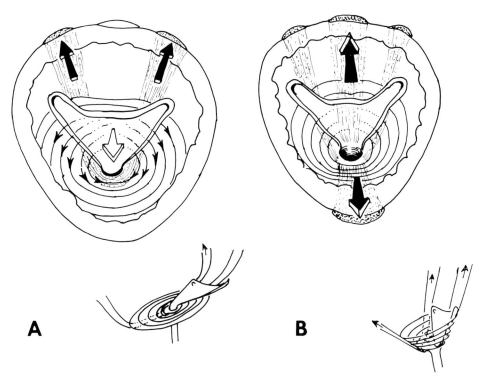

Figure I-16 A–B. Bladder filling. A., fundus ring pulls trigone forward against detrusor loop, closing bladder outlet; B., at micturition, the outermost anterior and posterior groups open the internal sphincter.

This controls the flow of blood into the organ. Upon erotic stimulation, the parasympathetic nervous system (S2, 3, 4) inhibits the tonic contraction of the helicine arteries, allowing blood to fill the cavernous sinusoids (until expansion of the organ is limited by the connective tissue tunica albuginea) and the penis becomes erect. Penile erection is under parasympathetic reflex control as is bladder emptying, with nerve fibers originating in S2, 3, 4. Sympathetics control both emission of semen from the ducts into the urethra and closure of the internal sphincter of the bladder. The pudendal nerve innervates the bulbocavernosus muscle which rhythmically contracts to propel semen from the urethra (ejaculation). Following orgasm, the sympathetic nervous system re-establishes tonic contraction of the helicine arteries, blood flow to the penis is reduced, and the engorged sinusoids are slowly drained by the veins.

The female urethra is 2.0 to 3.0 cm long. Changes in epithelial type closely parallel those of the male organ. The lamina propria also is similar, except that it is provided with a highly developed venous plexus resembling the corpus spongiosum of the male. The muscularis, with inner longitudinal and outer circular layers, is strengthened at the urogenital diaphragm by a sphincter of striated muscle.

The female urethra is enclosed in the anterior wall of the vagina, rather than in the clitoris, which is the female homologue of the penis (Plate I-7). Both urethra and vagina open into a space called the vestibule of the vagina, with the urethral orifice lying immediately anterior to that of the vagina. Enclosing the vestibule on either side are the labia minora and, lateral to these, the labia majora, covered with skin and pubic hair. Anteriorly lie the clitoris and mons pubis. The female external genitals collectively are called the vulva.

Both the vagina and urethra are slightly anterior to the anus so that fecal organisms can readily move into the vestibule and thence through the very short female urethra to the bladder, making the female bladder much more subject to infection than is the male bladder. Damage to the muscles of the urogenital diaphragm (as in childbirth or surgical procedures) may lead to incontinence in the female. Unfortunately, the anatomy of the vulva makes an external collecting device very difficult to design.

Venous and Lymphatic Drainage of the Pelvic Organs

The venous and lymphatic drainage of pelvic organs is rather complex and has implications for the spread of infection or metastasis.

In general, an anastomosing plexus of veins surrounds the bladder, prostate, vagina, and rectum (Plate I-9). Blood, upon leaving the plexuses, drains into either the internal iliac vessels or into the vertebral venous plexus. Two exceptions to this rule are the upper part of the rectum, which drains into the portal system by way of the superior rectal vein, and the upper uterine drainage, which may move through the uterine and ovarian plexuses and ovarian veins into the inferior vena cava on the right and the renal vein on the left. Drainage through the vertebral plexus may reach the azygos system and the superior vena cava.

Lymphatic drainage is also mixed (Plate I-10), with lymphatics from some superficial structures such as the external genitalia reaching superficial inguinal and external iliac nodes, while the more deeply lying organs drain into external iliac, internal iliac, and sacral nodes. Lymph nodes lie in series, and lymphatic vessels will usually drain through several nodes before reaching lumbar nodes lying alongside the aorta and inferior vena cava. From these nodes, large vessels called lumbar trunks flow into the cysterna chyli (just inferior to the diaphragm on the posterior abdominal wall) and from this through the thoracic duct into the left subclavian vein in the neck.

Again, the exception to this organization is the upper rectum which drains through mesenteric nodes into the cysterna chyli.

PATHOLOGY OF THE URINARY SYSTEM

Introduction

Individuals with neurological diseases or defects will often exhibit dysfunction of the urinary tract. Disorders of the brain such as Parkinson's disease, dementia, cerebral vascular accident, or brain tumors frequently produce urinary tract symptoms as do spinal cord injury, spinal malformations or tumors, intervertebral disk problems, vascular accidents of the cord, and changes that accompany aging. Other diseases which can affect bladder function are multiple sclerosis, pernicious anemia, pelvic surgery or carcinoma of pelvic organs, poliomyelitis, and diabetes. There are, of course, others.

Neurogenic Bladder

Neurogenic (neuropathic) bladder is a name given to disorder of the bladder innervation, often secondary to other neurological defects.[9, 19-21] A neurogenic bladder is the result of interruption of normal neural control of the bladder by trauma or disease. In infants, the involuntary or automatic reflex emptying of the bladder takes place through the spinal cord levels S2, 3, and 4. Stretch sensors in the bladder wall send impulses through the pelvic nerves to the spinal cord where they synapse with the parasympathetic neurons which stimulate bladder contraction, and inhibit the pudendal nerve, resulting in the relaxation of the external sphincter.

Normally, volunary voiding of urine is controlled by the brain through nerve fibers running in spinal cord tracts to S2, 3 and 4 levels where they modulate both the parasympathetic (pelvic nerves) and somatic (pudendal nerves) outflow.

When a cord injury or disease of the central nervous system occurs above the S2,3,4 levels, volitional control of the bladder is lost resulting in an *"automatic (reflex) neurogenic bladder"* which empties itself reflexly (Fig. I-17).

Injury to the sacral levels of the cord or peripheral nerves which arise there (pelvic, pudendal) abolishes the reflex involved in micturition so that the bladder will empty only by overflowing. This is called an *"autonomous neurogenic bladder"* (Fig. I-18).

Partial denervation may result in *dyssynergia* (an uncoordinated bladder and external sphincter) or weak bladder contractions. Complications of

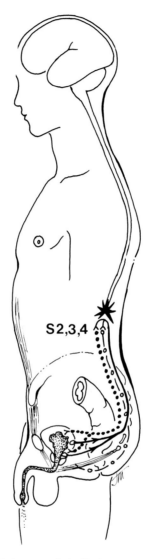

S2,3,4

Figure I-17. Autonomic (reflex) neurogenic bladder.

renal function which arise as a result of neurogenic bladder may be prevented or ameliorated by proper long-term care.

We will discuss the neurogenic bladder in the long-term care of the patient afflicted with neurologic disease or disorder, as well as some conditions primarily affecting the urinary tract that present significant problems in the care of these individuals. For a more complete discussion of specific neurological diseases and the urinary tract, the reader may consult pathology texts.[9,22,23]

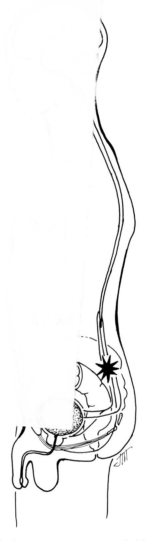

Figure I-18. Autonomous neurogenic bladder.

Obstructive and Constrictive Uropathy

To understand the mechanism of disease secondary to obstruction, it is helpful to review the anatomy of the urinary tract. Urine drips from the collecting ducts of the kidney into the minor calyces, cup-like structures which are confluent with the major calyces and renal pelvis. The funnel-shaped pelvis narrows to become the ureter at the inferior pole of the kidney (called the ureteropelvic junction), courses retroperitoneally over the pelvic brim, and enters the posterosuperior aspect of the bladder wall in an anteromedial direction (Fig. I-19). The intramural course of the ureter is oblique. The ureteropelvic junction where the renal pelvis narrows (Fig. I-19A), the pelvic brim where the ureter is bent over the common iliac vessels (Fig. I-19B), and the intramural course of the ureter are all potential sites of obstruction (Fig. I-19C). In addition, the bladder outlet may be compressed by a hypertrophied prostate or tumor (Fig. I-19D). Acquired obstructions of the bladder outlet include *strictures* of the urethra as a result of infection or injury, *benign prostatic hyperplasia* or *cancer of the prostate*, and cancers of the prostate or cervix which extend to the bladder and occlude the ureteral orifices (Fig. I-19E). The bladder itself may be the site of tumors which obstruct the bladder neck or the ureteral orifices, and metastatic nodes may compress the ureter at the pelvic brim. *Ureteral stones (calculi)* may lodge in the ureter or pelvis and obstruct the free movement of urine. Retroperitoneal malignancy, pregnancy, and severe constipation (especially in children) may also compress the ureter. Finally, a neurogenic bladder may have the same effect on the upper urinary tract as any of the above obstructions because of its inability to empty effectively.

Distal (urethral) obstructions result in hypertrophy of the bladder muscle as it attempts to expel urine past the obstruction.[9] Bundles of smooth muscle form thick ridges called *trabeculae* which are interspersed with increased amounts of connective tissue, apparently elaborated by the smooth muscle cells. Hypertrophy of the trigone causes increased resistance to urine flow in the intramural ureter due to accentuated downward pull on the muscle involved in the ureterovesical junction. Significant residual urine volume increases the traction on trigonal muscle with the same effect. The increased vesical pressures required to force urine from the obstructed bladder may also force mucosal pockets called *cellules* between the trabeculated muscle bundles (Fig. I-20). If these are pushed entirely through the bladder wall they are called *diverticula*. They have no muscle in their walls and fail to expel residual urine efficiently, leading to stasis and infection which is difficult to eradicate.

With trabeculation of the bladder, *intravesical pressure* is increased during the act of voiding. At first the ureterovesical junction prevents the pressure from being transmitted to ureters and kidneys. Recall that the bladder musculature spirals around the intramural ureter and that detrusor (bladder muscle) contraction effects closure of the intramural lumen. At the same time urine is prevented from flowing freely into the bladder, and for this reason there is progessive back pressure on the ureter and kidney from urine accumulating in the ureter. This leads eventually to dilation of the ureter (*hydroureter*) (Fig. I-21), renal pelvis and calyces (*hydronephrosis*). Continuing obstruction of the urethra will cause the bladder muscle to

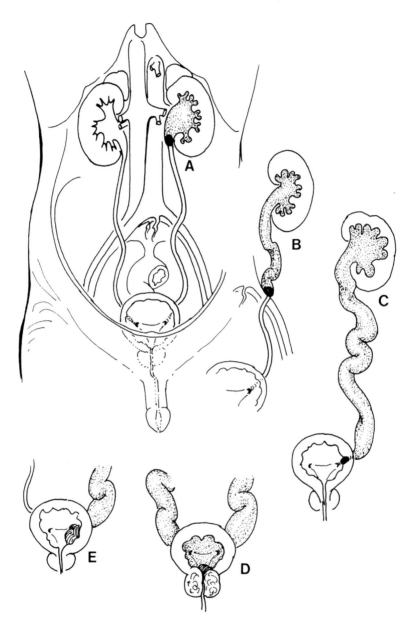

Figure I-19. Obstructive or constrictive uropathy results in back pressure on ureter and kidney from accumulation of urine in ureter. A. Stone lodged at ureteropelvic junction. B. Stone lodged at iliac vessels. C. Intramural stone. D. Hypertrophied prostate gland obstructing urethra. E. Bladder tumor obstructing ureterovesical junction.

decompensate and become less effective in expelling urine, with residual urine remaining in the bladder (*stasis*) after voiding. This encourages the

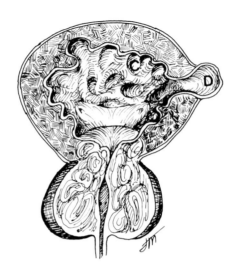

Figure I-20. Urethral obstruction results in bladder trabeculation and formation of cellules (C) and diverticula (D).

growth of bacteria and infection of the bladder wall (*cystitis*). In decompensation the ureterovesical mechanism may lose its valve-like action, allowing the increased intravesical pressure to be transmitted to the ureter and renal pelvis. Urine may be forced up into the ureters from the bladder (*vesicoureteral reflux, VUR*), carrying infection, if present, with it.[24,25]

Back pressure on the ureters leads to hypertrophy of ureteral musculature as it attempts to force urine into the bladder by increased peristalsis. Ultimately, in the face of increased pressures, the ureter, too, decompensates and loses its contractile power. Dilation may be extreme and the ureter tortuous.

Upper tract obstruction may be caused by kidney stones arrested in passage through the ureter at the sites where the organ narrows. This results in back pressure as they prevent the passage of urine through the system. We have had several patients with neurogenic bladders in which partial obstruction at the ureteropelvic junction by blood vessels has caused pelvic dilatation.

The renal pelvis may lie entirely within the renal sinus or may be largely extrarenal. Normally, pressure within is close to zero. As the pressure increases due to vesicoureteral reflux or obstruction, the pelvis hypertrophies and expands. If it lies outside the kidney, much of the pressure may be dissipated. However, an *intrarenal pelvis* transmits pressure directly to the kidney parenchyma, with a limited amount being absorbed by the bed of fat in which the pelvis lies. Infection of the pelvis (*pyelitis*) may result from organisms ascending from the bladder by way of vesicoureteral reflux.

In the kidney early damage from hydronephrosis is seen at the minor

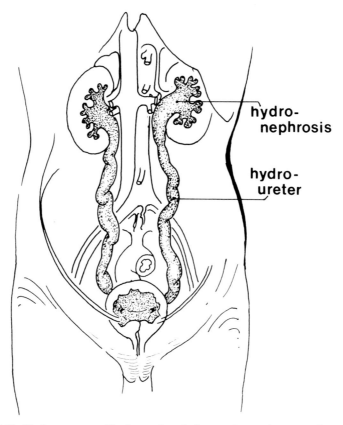

Figure I-21. Hydroureter and hydronephrosis due to obstructive uropathy.

calyx. The papilla of the medullary pyramid projects into the calyx producing *fornices* which sharply define the concavity of the calyx. Initially, calyces respond to increased pressure by hypertrophy of the muscle in their walls. With sustained increases in intrapelvic pressures, the fornices become rounded (*calyceal blunting*) and the papilla is compressed and flattened (Fig. I-19C). The expanding pelvis also compresses the blood vessels (between the centrally increasing pressure and the inflexible renal capsule) resulting in parenchymal atrophy secondary to ischemia. Increased pressures are also transmitted to the collecting ducts and tubules, and their cells are similarly affected.

The movement of urine in a retrograde direction from bladder to kidney (reflux) may have a number of causes.[24,25] Congenital weakness at the ureterovesical junction or ureteral abnormalities account for some cases. Spastic neurogenic bladder or severe distal obstruction associated with trabeculation and trigonal hypertrophy may cause a diverticulum through the ureteral hiatus and a resultant lack of muscle to occlude the opening.

Edema of the vesical wall secondary to cystitis may impair valvular function. It is also possible that surgical intervention such as prostatectomy or wedge resection of the posterior vesical neck may cause sufficient damage to the trigonal muscle to make the valve incompetent.

Hydroureteronephrosis is usually associated with reflux because of increased workload (urine moving both up and down the tract), increased hydrostatic pressure causing stretching and dilation, and weakened ureteral musculature. The ureteropelvic and ureterovesical junctions are less distensible than the rest of the ureter and may not be able to pass normal urine plus refluxed urine, resulting in functional obstruction. Even sterile reflux can damage the kidney, as the presence of extravasated urine in the kidney interstitium elicits an inflammatory response with fibrosis and scarring of the parenchyma.

Pyelonephritis

Pyelonephritis most often is a complication of vesicoureteral reflux. It is a bacterial infection of kidney parenchyma which has usually ascended by way of reflux of contaminated urine from an infected bladder.[26,27] Bacteria may also reach the kidney through the bloodstream, though obstruction seems necessary to the development of pyelonephritis. The organisms in ascending infection are frequently *E. coli*, *Proteus*, *Klebsiella* or *Pseudomonas*, and the signs they produce include fever, flank pain (in the neurologically intact individual), white blood cells in the urine, casts, urgency, and frequency. Pyelonephritis is a tubulointerstitial disease in which the acute inflammatory response ruptures into the tubules. The cortex of the kidney may exhibit microabscesses and the tubules may be destroyed. Histologically, there is evidence of acute inflammation with mononuclear cell infiltration, formation of fibrous tissue, and asymmetric renal scarring. Pyelonephritis may become chronic in the absence of prompt and adequate treatment, particularly if vesicoureteral reflux is present. Glomeruli and tubules show varying degrees of involvement, and blood vessels become thickened. Symptoms are few, although mild discomfort over the kidney, vesical irritability, and hypertension may be present. If treatment is delayed, the kidney may become badly scarred and atrophied.

Benign Prostatic Hyperplasia

The prostate enlarges with age; 80 percent of octogenarians have an enlarged prostate with urinary obstruction. Called *benign prostatic hyperplasia (BPH)*, this enlargement is hormonally related, although the cause is not entirely clear. As the gland enlarges, it begins to occlude the prostatic urethra and to interfere with the action of the internal sphincter of the bladder, creating increased resistance to the passage of urine. In response to urethral constriction, the bladder hypertrophies and becomes trabeculated and diverticula are formed. Later, the bladder decompensates, urine is retained, and vesicoureteral reflux, hydoureter, and upper tract infection ensue. Three lobes of the gland are commonly involved in hyperplasia and may herniate through the bladder neck. A "surgical capsule" made up of compressed prostate is poorly attached to the central hyperplastic nodules and often allows enucleation of the obstructing tissue with relief of the urethral constriction.

Aminoglycoside Nephrotoxicity

Aminoglycoside antibiotics (e.g. amikacin, tobramycin, neomycin, gentamicin) may produce a variety of abnormalities ranging from decreased output of urine to complete loss of kidney function with uremia.[28,29] They are the most common cause of drug-induced acute renal failure, accounting for 10 percent of all such cases of that disease.

At the cellular level, there is damage to the plasma membrane of the cell and its organelles with changes in the phospholipid content of the membranes and alterations in cell permeability and transport. The glomerulus and proximal tubule are affected early; the distal tubule later. There appears to be a net reabsorption of aminoglycoside along the proximal tubule, with accumulation primarily in the parenchyma of the cortex. In the glomerulus, the endothelial cells swell and there is a decrease in size and number of the fenestrae which results in decreased glomerular filtration. The cells of the proximal tubule exhibit increased numbers of secondary lysosomes with myelin figures, perhaps representing autophagia of damaged organelles. Later, there is necrosis and desquamation of the epithelium and cytoplasmic debris in the tubular lumen. In the medulla there is injury to the loop of Henle and collecting duct, with interstitial fibrosis and scarring sufficient to produce papillary necrosis.

The toxic effects on the urinary tract include concentrating defects which produce polyuria and nephrogenic diabetes insipidus because the drug inhibits antidiuretic hormone.

Among predisposing factors, dose and duration of drug administration are most important. Higher doses result in more rapid accumulation of the toxin in the kidney, while prolonged therapy achieves toxic concentrations. Recent or repeated aminoglycoside therapy increases the risk. When the drugs are withdrawn, most of the mild cases will recover. There is regeneration of the tubules, but focal scarring may often be seen in the cortex.

Polycystic Disease

Renal polycystic disease is a congenital, bilateral disease which may be divided into autosomal recessive (infantile type) and autosomal dominant (affecting primarily persons in the 30–60 year age range). It may be caused by a defect of development of some of the uriniferous tubules, perhaps the non-union of distal convoluted tubule and collecting duct. Cysts, which are seen in the cortex and medulla of the kidney, enlarge, exert pressure on the surrounding parenchyma, and result in its destruction. Bleeding into the cysts may produce hematuria. Uremia develops very slowly.

Associated with polycystic disease are cysts of liver (dilated bile ducts) and pancreas, as well as hypertension and aneurysm of the cerebral circle of Willis. In the adult, polycystic disease may also be complicated by pyelonephritis or renal tumors.

Amyloidosis

Amyloidosis is characterized by extracellular accumulations of a fine fibrillar protein, amyloid, in deposits beneath the endothelium of capillaries and sinusoids.[22,23,30] It is associated with the glomerular capillaries of the kidney cortex and may accumulate to the extent that it obliterates the glomerulus. Microscopically, there is fusion of podocyte foot processes, which probably interferes with ultrafiltration.

Symptoms include hypertension, proteinuria, edema, and progressive deterioration of renal function. The individual is susceptible to infection and thromboembolism due to an increase in the synthesis of clotting factors secondary to proteinuria.

Hypertension

The kidney has a dual role in hypertension.[31-33] Its prohypertensive effect is controlled by the renin-angiotensin mechanism and/or the expansion of the extracellular fluid volume and plasma volume due to the effects of aldosterone. Antihypertensive effects may be the result of renomedullary interstitial cells which synthesize prostaglandins, vasodilators which produce diuresis and sodium excretion.[34]

Vessels of the kidney react to hypertension with thickened walls and narrowed lumens. The mesangium thickens as a result of increased capillary pressures. Microinfarcts cause a loss of parenchyma due to ischemia, while red cells may be broken in the narrowed vessels, resulting in microangiopathic hemolytic anemia.

Hypertension is associated with narrowing of the renal artery as well, which means that the blood reaches the juxtaglomerular apparatus at a reduced pressure. As a consequence, renin is released, causing increased blood pressure in the body as a whole in order to deliver blood at the correct perfusion pressure to the kidney.

Neoplasm

Neoplasm is new, pathologic growth of tissue which may be either malignant or benign. If *malignant,* growth is irregular and produces an atypical, unencapsulated structure which infiltrates the surrounding tissues. The cells are poorly differentiated and undergo frequent abnormal mitosis. Metastasis to other tissues and organs takes place. A *benign* neoplasm lacks these characteristics but may be injurious or fatal to the host if its growth impinges on adjacent structures and impairs their function.

Neoplasms of the kidney are primarily of two varieties.[22,23] Renal cell adenocarcinoma, apparently deriving from the renal tubules, accounts for about 80 percent of renal malignancies, while transitional cell carcinoma of the calyces, pelvis and ureters, probably caused by carcinogens, comprises 5 percent to 10 percent of them. Fever, weight loss, fatigue, flank pain, hematuria, anemia and hypertension are symptoms of renal malignancy. However, the first signs may be caused by metastases. Neurologic symptoms are produced by hematogenous spread to spinal cord and brain, while metastasis to liver produces jaundice; to lungs, pleuritic pain; and to lymph nodes, effects secondary to enlargement of the nodes such as edema of the legs or functional obstruction of the ureters. Benign tumors of the kidney are rare.

Bladder carcinoma arises from transitional epithelial cells which become atypical and show a loss of polarity. Lesions are seen mostly in the lateral walls and trigone and may cause blockage of the ureters. If the tumor invades the muscular wall of the bladder, it may metastasize to the surrounding lymph nodes. Invasion of perineural areas will cause pain.

Urinary tract infections, obstruction, and stones are associated with *squamous metaplasia* which is thought to be a reaction to chronic irritation. Patients who are managed with indwelling catheters for many years are subject to squamous metaplasia or transitional cell carcinoma of the bladder and urethra.[35] Incidence increases with duration of catheterization. Hematuria associated with these changes may be gross but is often microscopic, and lesions may not be visible endoscopically. The presence of infection, which may be almost universal in these patients, is not considered diagnostic.

Cancer of the prostate makes up 16 percent of all primary malignancies in males and usually causes urinary obstruction. Metastasis to surrounding tissues occurs frequently with spread to skeletal tissues.

SUMMARY

In this chapter we have described briefly the functional anatomy of the normal human urinary system and some of the diseases and malfunctions to which it is prone in the context of the chronically disabled individual. This in no way constitutes a comprehensive list of the diseases of the urinary system but, instead, discusses malfunctions commonly encountered in long-term care of the disabled. In the chapters to follow we will deal in some detail with these problems and suggest ways of coping with them.

J.M.

REFERENCES

1. Farquhar, Marilyn G.: The role of the basement membrane in glomerular filtration: Results obtained with electron-dense tracers. In Maunsbach, A. (Ed.): *Functional Ultrastructure of the Kidney.* London, Academic Press, 1981.
2. Farquhar, Marilyn G.: The glomerular basement membrane—a selective macromolecular filter. In Hay, Elizabeth D. (Ed.): *Cell Biology of the Extracellular Matrix.* New York, Plenum, 1981.
3. Karnovsky, Morris J.: The structural basis for glomerular filtration. In Churg, Jacob (Ed.): *Kidney Disease: Present Status.* Baltimore, Williams and Wilkins, 1979.
4. Venkatachalam, Manjeri; and Rennke, Helmut, G.: Glomerular filtration of macromolecules: Structural, molecular, and functional determinants. In Leaf, A. (Ed.): *Renal Pathophysiology.* New York, Raven Press, 1980.
5. Wolgast, Hermanson, Nygren, Larson, and Sjoquist: The glomerular ultrafiltration process. In Maunsbach, A. (Ed.): *Functional Ultrastructure of the Kidney.* London, Academic Press, 1980.
6. Severs, N.J., and Hicks, R.M.: Analysis of membrane structure in the transitional epithelium of rat urinary bladder. *J Ultrastruct Res 69:*279–296, 1979.
7. Weiss, Robert M., Bassett, A.L., and Hoffman, Brian: Adrenergic innervation of the ureter. *Invest Urol 16:*2:123–127, 1978.
8. Elbadawi, Ahmed: Anatomy and function of the ureteral sheath. *J Urol 102:*224–229, 1972.
9. Hald, Tage, and Bradley, William E.: *The Urinary Bladder: Neurology and Dynamics.* Baltimore, Williams and Wilkins, 1982.
10. Elbadawi, Ahmed; and Schenk, Eric A.: A new theory of the innervation of the bladder musculature, Part 3: Post-ganglionic synapses in uretero-vesical-urethral autonomic pathways. *J Urol 105:*372–374, 1971.
11. Elbadawi, Ahmed; and Schenk, Eric A.: A new theory of the innervation of bladder musculature, Part 4: Innervation of vesicourethral junction and external urethral sphincter. *J Urol 111:*613–615, 1974.
12. Hoffman, Brian B., and Lefkowitz, R.J.: Alpha adrenergic receptor subtypes, *N Engl J Med 302:*1390–1396, 1980.
13. Nergardh, Arne: Autonomic receptor functions in the lower urinary tract: A survey of recent experimental results. *J Urol 113:*180–185, 1975.
14. Sundin, Torsten; Dahlstrom, A.; Norlen, L.; and Svedmyr, N.: The sympathetic innervation

and adrenoreceptor function in the human lower urinary tract in the normal state and after parasympathetic denervation. *Invest Urol 14:4:*322–328, 1977.

15. Tulloch, Alastair, G.S.: Sympathetic activity of internal urethral sphincter. *Urol 5:3:*353–355, 1975.

16. deGroat, William C., and Booth, A.M.: Inhibition and facilitation in parasympathetic ganglia of the urinary bladder. *Fed Proc 39:*2990–2996, 1980.

17. Koyanagi, Tomohiko: Studies on the sphincteric system located distally in the urethra: The external urethral sphincter revisited. *J Urol 124:*400–406, 1980.

18. Hutch, John A.: *The Anatomy and Physiology of the Bladder, Trigone, and Urethra.* New York, Appleton-Century-Crofts, 1972.

19. Boyarsky, Saul: *Care of the Patient with Neurogenic Bladder.* 1st ed. Boston, Little Brown, 1979.

20. Koff, S.A., Diokno, A.C., and Lapides, J.: Neurogenic bladder dysfunction. *Am Fam Physician 19:*100–109, 1979.

21. McGuire, Edward J.: *Clinical Evaluation and Treatment of Neurogenic Vesical Dysfunction.* Baltimore, Williams and Wilkins, 1984.

22. Robbins, S.L., Cotran, R.S., and Kumar, V.: *Pathologic Basis of Disease.* 3rd ed. Philadelphia, W.B. Saunders Co, 1984.

23. Smith, Lloyd H. Jr., and Thier, Samual O.: *Pathophysiology: The Biological Principles of Disease.* Vol. 1. International Textbook of Medicine. Edited by Samiy, Smith and Wyngaarden. Philadelphia, W.B. Saunders, 1981.

24. Libertino, John A.: Adult vesicoureteral reflux. In J. Herbert Johnston (Ed.): *Management of Vesicoureteral Reflux.* Baltimore, Williams and Wilkins, 1984.

25. Salvatierra, Oscar; and Tanagho, Emil: Reflux as a cause of end stage kidney disease: A report of 32 cases. *J Urol 117:*441–443, 1977.

26. Cotran, Ramzi S.: Interstitial nephritis. In Churg, Jacob (Ed.): *Kidney Disease: Present Status.* Baltimore, Williams and Wilkins, 1979.

27. Kory, Michael; and Waife, S.O.: *Kidney and Urinary Tract Infections.* Indianapolis, Lilly Research Laboratories, 1971.

28. Humes, H. David, Weinberg, Joel M., and Knauss, T.C.: Clinical and pathophysiologic aspects of aminoglycoside nephrotoxicity. *Am J Kidney Disease 2:*5–29, 1982.

29. Weinstein, Louis; and Weinstein, Allen J.: The pathophysiology and pathoanatomy of reactions to antimicrobial agents. *Adv Inter Med 19:*109–128, 1974.

30. Cohen, Alan S., and Cathcart, Edgar S.: Amyloidosis and immunoglobulins. *Adv Intern Med 19:*41–52, 1974.

31. Kaplan, Norman M.: Renal dysfunction in essential hypertension. *N Engl J Med 309:*1052, 1983.

32. Muirhead, E.E.: The role of the renal medulla in hypertension. *Adv Intern Med 19:*81–101, 1974.

33. Curtis, John J.: Remission of essential hypertension after renal transplantation. *N Engl J Med 309:*1009–1015, 1983.

34. Bohman, Sven-Olof: The ultrastructure and function of the interstitial cells of the renal medulla, with special regard to prostaglandin synthesis. In Maunsbach, A. (Ed.): *Functional Ultrastructure of the Kidney.* London, Academic Press, 1980.

35. Kaufman, G.M., Fam, B., Jacobs, S.C., Gabilondo, F., Yalla, S., Kane, G.P., and Rossier, A.B.: Bladder cancer and squamous metaplasia in spinal cord injured patients. *J Urol 118:*967–971, 1977.

36. Anderson, G.F., and Marks, B.H.: Spare cholinergic receptors in the urinary bladder. *J Pharmacol Exp Ther 221:*598–603, 1982.

37. Anderson, G.F., and Marks, B.H.: Beta adrenergic receptors in the rabbit bladder and detrusor muscle. *J Pharmacol Exp Ther* 228:2:283–286, 1984.
38. Gilmore, Joseph P.: *Renal Physiology.* Baltimore, Williams and Wilkins, 1972.
39. Lote, Christopher J.: *Principles of Renal Physiology.* London, Croom Helm Ltd., 1982.
40. Pirani, C.L., and Silva, F.G.: The glomerulus: Current concepts. In Remuzzi, Mecca, and de Gaetano (Eds.): *Homeostasis, Prostaglandins, and Renal Disease.* New York, Raven Press, 1980.
41. Plum, Fred; and Colfelt, Robert H.: The genesis of vesical rhythmicity. *Arch Neurol, AMA* 2:487–496, 1960.
42. Raezer, David M., Greenberg, S.H., Jacobowitz, D.M., Benson, G.S., Corriere, Jr., J.N., and Wein, Alan J.: Innervation of the trigonal area of canine urinary bladder. *Urol* 7:369–375, 1976.
43. Smith, D.R.: *General Urology.* 10th ed. Los Altos, Lange Medical Publications, 1981.

Chapter II

PRINCIPLES OF TREATMENT OF THE DISABLED BLADDER

GOALS

B efore the treatment of any condition can be successful, certain particulars must be clear:

1. The goals of therapy.
2. Obstacles to goal achievement.
3. The most effective method to achieve the goal.

The *principle aim* in the care of the disabled bladder is to preserve kidney function. It has been said that the bladder is a social organ but that the kidneys are a matter of life and death. Certainly, the kidneys are of utmost importance in influencing water balance, protein and carbohydrate metabolism, hematopoiesis, and blood pressure control; nonetheless, it must be recognized that in addition to controlling urine expulsion, the bladder serves as a guardian of the kidneys, preventing ascent of infection and modifying the fluctuation of hydraulic pressure to the upper tracts.

A *second goal* of treatment is the maintenance of the social acceptability of the disabled person by eliminating wetness of skin, clothing and furniture and preventing a pervasive urinary odor.

A *third objective* entails keeping the drudgery of bladder care to a minimum so that patient and attendants will not become so discouraged and frustrated that they neglect essentials. In order to accomplish the latter goal, all involved persons must understand the relationships of the caretaking tasks to the primary and secondary goals, securing the proper equipment for performing the tasks and organizing procedures so that they can be executed in an efficient and routine manner.

DETERRENTS TO GOAL ACHIEVEMENT

There are *cognitive, psychological and physical obstacles* to the accomplishment of such objectives. Lack of knowledge of the anatomy of the urinary tract as well as the effects of pathologic processes upon its function is one of the greatest hindrances to optimal care. Chapter I deals with this subject in

43

detail and merits careful study. Briefly, the neurologically impaired bladder does not have the defenses of the normal bladder for preventing infection, overdistention, and urine stagnation. A knowledgeable and conscientious team comprised of the patient, the attendants and the other health care providers can usually compensate for these inadequacies but only by accepting the responsibilities for ongoing, systematic daily care.

A second hazard is that of decreasing motivation. The initial enthusiasm for care provision can be dulled by fatigue, lack of appreciation, and the intrusion of life's other trials. It is imperative that health care professionals be sensitive to the development of these factors and be willing to provide support in combatting them by reinforcing the knowledge that daily, meticulous care is essential in preventing infections, stone formation, reflux and kidney failure and that only the people providing these services can ensure such results.

A third danger is the eagerness to grasp at the "latest" fashion in treatment without complete knowledge of its appropriateness to the involved person's disability. Changes in care should be made only after careful consideration, including consultation with professionals who have had experience with the proposed methods.

In addition to psychosocial deterrents, *pathological complications* may hinder goal achievement (e.g. infection, bladder overdistention, calculus formation, reflux, obstruction, dyssynergia and autonomic dysreflexia). Such conditions will be dealt with in detail later.

Often overlooked in the plan for bladder care are the *environmental and financial circumstances* of the patient. A low income person living on an Indian reservation will not have the facilities for self-care enjoyed by a moderate income individual in a city apartment. While the highest possible standards should be maintained, it must be kept in mind that a simple routine systematically performed will produce better results than a highly technical regimen only occasionally employed.

METHODS FOR ACHIEVING GOALS

Methods for achieving the goals of preservation of renal function, maintenance of social acceptability, and the efficient use of patient and attendant energies are influenced by the selection of the *proper mode of urinary tract drainage.*[1] This choice is best made by conference among health care providers, attendants and patient. Each can contribute unique and relevant information regarding the current and changing degree of disability, difficulties of equipment care, and the esthetic appeal of the available methods. Flexibility in planning is essential. With the passing of time, conditions may change, making different methods desirable. The most frequently used methods of drainage are intermittent catheterization, the appliance free state often aided by physical stimulation or by suprapubic pressure (Crede), external catheter drainage with or without stimulation or pressure, indwelling urethral catheterization, indwelling suprapubic catheterization, and urinary diversion.

Indwelling catheter use is now less frequently necessary because of improved methods of treatment of the disabled bladder in its early stages.

Ileal or colonic diversion has been largely replaced by other methods of treatment, although it is occasionally a lifesaving procedure.

The use of the external catheter has been facilitated by several surgical procedures. The development of external sphincterotomy to overcome outflow resistance often produces a residual-free bladder. As electronic techniques are improved, electrical bladder stimulation should more frequently prove beneficial to those with lower motor neurone bladders. Penile prostheses have been used to assist in the use of external catheters in male patients with small genitalia. Good results are frequent, but the patient should be aware of the complications which may develop with each type of prosthetic implant.

Males using external drainage and females using catheters can sometimes be made appliance-free through the use of the artificial sphincter. Its utilization will undoubtedly be increased as technical development makes possible more precise control of sphincter closing pressure. At present, its use must be cautiously considered, especially by those with sensory deficits. The development of pressure sores with urethral erosion is not infrequent and can be catastrophic, particularly in women.

Intermittent catheterization has proved a useful technique in the management of the disabled bladder. With sudden onset of bladder dysfunction, its use can avoid overdistention and infection until function spontaneously resumes. During hospitalized management of such conditions as spinal cord injury, success is directly proportional to the degree of cooperation among medical personnel, nursing staff and the patient, if he/she is able to cooperate. Fluid intake and periodicity of catheterization must be carefully manipulated to avoid overdistention. Scrupulous techniques must be observed to avoid nosocomial infections.[2]

Post-hospital-discharge use of intermittent catheterization has been successful in the hands of many. Lapides[3] states that if fluids are controlled and the bladder is emptied every three hours, infection and overdistention need not be feared. We have found it very difficult to enforce an every-three-hour emptying regimen, especially if the patient is working or going to school. Even with the use of a meticulously clean technique of catheterization, infection has been a problem. With dirty techniques it has been a greater problem. Our best results have been with males with good hand function whose motivation has been great enough to restrict fluids, empty the bladder regularly and maintain a cleanly technique. While some women with the same qualifications have been successful, they have had more difficulty remaining dry between emptying and in finding accessible toilets.

After decisions about urinary tract drainage have been made, the *volume and timing of fluid intake* must be selected. This is relatively easy for patients with indwelling urethral catheters, suprapubic catheters, and urinary diversions, because obstruction to outflow is not a problem in properly functioning systems. In such patients the chief concern is with providing sufficient bladder or conduit washout to remove bacteria while ensuring water intake volumes which will maintain fluid balance. Usually 2000 ml to 3000 ml per day in divided doses is adequate.

With other methods of drainage which do not have continuous outflow of urine from the body, more thought must be given to total volume and to periodicity of intake so that bladder distention can be avoided. Enough fluid must be taken to provide adequate washout several times a day without ingesting so much that overdistention results from slight prolongation of daytime emptying intervals, from the longer periods of non-emptying during sleeping hours, or the diuresis due to psychologic, pharmacologic, or physical factors. These problems will be discussed at length in Chapter IV.

In summary, adequate fluid intake, the proper choice of urinary tract drainage plus meticulous hygiene will usually assure good urinary tract function, but occasionally complications arise due to unnoticed non-compliance, accidental obstruction to outflow, or changed pathophysiology beyond the control of patient and health care providers. The most common complications are infection, obstruction to outflow, increasing residual urine, stones, detrusor-sphincter dyssynergia, autonomic dysreflexia, reflux, and kidney failure.

It is important that the patient and all personnel involved in his care be aware of the signs and symptoms of such complications and that intra-team communication be free flowing. If, for any reason, the usual channels of communication are unavailable, each member of the team should feel free to contact the physicians whenever problems arise.

M.P.

REFERENCES

1. Abramson, A.: Management of the neurogenic bladder in perspective. *Arch Phys Med Rehabil* 57:197–201, 1976.

2. Guttman, L.: Management of paralysis, intermittent catheterization. *Brit Surg Pract 6:*445, 1949.
3. Lapides, J., Diokno, A., Silber, S., and Lowe, B.: Clean, intermittent self-catheterization in the treatment of urinary tract disease. *J Urol 107:*458, 1972.

Chapter III

INFECTION—THE PROCESS AND ETIOLOGY

When considering infections we are concerned not only with the recognition of the organisms involved but also the nature of illness and the principles of treatment, prevention and control. These are similar for all infections. To understand the principles of infection control, it is important to understand the factors affecting the ability of the microorganism to produce an infectious disease and the ability of the host to resist disease.

MICROORGANISM—HOST RELATIONSHIPS

There are several relationships which may exist between the microorganism and the host.

Independent: Microorganisms may live side by side with the host completely independent of each other.

Commencialism: The microorganism and the host may live together in a symbiotic manner with one or both benefitting and with no harm to the other. An example of this is the resident or normal flora of the skin.

Mutualism: Both the host and the microorganism benefit from this form of symbiosis. An example is the normal microflora of the intestinal tract.

Parasitism: The host and microorganism live together in a symbiotic relationship with one benefitting at the expense of the other. If the microorganism is benefitting at the expense of the host, an infectious disease results.

The relationship between microorganism and host may change as conditions change. A bacterium living on the skin as normal flora (commencialism) may become parasitic if it enters into the tissue, grows, multiplies and spreads.

Precisely stated, *infection* is a state in which a host harbors microorganisms that survive and multiply in or on the tissue. An *infectious disease* is the manifestation of the infection and may be acute or chronic. In an *acute* infectious disease either the host or the microorganisms survive for a relatively short period of time, while in a *chronic* infectious disease, there is a prolonged relationship between the host and the microorganism. The term *infection* has come to be used interchangeably with *infectious disease* and has been used in that manner throughout this book.

What are the damaging properties of microorganisms that allow them to become parasitic upon the host? Several terms are used to describe these properties. *Pathogenicity* refers to the ability of the microbe to produce disease. *Virulence* is the degree of pathogenicity of the microorganism. Virulence can be measured experimentally by determining the minimum number of a given species of organism required to kill a specific test animal. This is referred to as the *minimum lethal dose* (MLD). *Invasiveness* refers to the ability of the microorganism to invade the host, multiply and spread and to protect itself from the host. The pathogenicity and virulence of an organism will depend upon its invasiveness and upon its *toxicity* or ability to produce substances that are harmful to the host cells and tissue.

Microorganisms may gain entry into the host in several ways: through the respiratory or gastrointestinal tract, mucosa, intact skin or by trauma or injection. Bacteria may be carried from the site of entry to other areas of the body through the circulatory or lymphatic systems.

HOST RESISTANCE

The human body has many specific and non-specific defense systems that help to resist infection.[1]

Non-Specific Resistance

Intact skin or *mucosa* serve as a barrier to most microorganisms. (An exception would be the spirochete causing syphilis.) The skin is protected by a tough layer of keratin which is a proteinaceous substance and by secretions from sebaceous and sweat glands. Mucous membranes may be protected by their secretions which trap particulate matter. The particulate matter is then removed by motile cell surface specializations called *cilia*, which sweep the mucous secretions out of the area.

Cellular and Fluid Elements

The blood plays an important role in the resistance to infection. The plasma (fluid portion of the blood) contains antibodies and complement which is necessary for the action of the antibodies. The cellular portion of the blood contains leukocytes or white blood cells which are capable of phagocytosis. These white cells are present at points of entry of a foreign object. They are able to migrate out of the capillaries and attack the foreign object, engulfing and digesting it. The action of these phagocytes is enhanced by other elements present in the plasma.

Mononuclear Phagocyte System

Lymphatic tissue is scattered throughout the body under surface epithelia and in nodes which are connected by lymphatic vessels. These nodes are lined with phagocytes that filter out bacterial cells. Lymphatic cells are also involved in the production of antibodies.

Inflammation

Inflammation is a body tissue response to infection or injury. It is usually characterized by redness, swelling and heat, and represents the reaction of the non-specific defense mechanism. The small blood vessels dilate and allow phagocytic cells to migrate through the vessel walls into the adjacent tissue. The phagocytic cells sometimes join together to form giant cells that wall off the foreign object (e.g. bacteria). Fluid and cells collect in the area of injury to form an *exudate*. If this exudate is thick and yellow and contains large numbers of leukocytes, it is called a *purulent exudate*. The exudate may also be *serous* (watery with fewer cells) or *fibrinous* (forming a clot). If the inflamed area becomes walled with fibrinous clots or connective tissue, an *abscess* results. The abscess may rupture and spread the infection to surrounding tissue, be surgically drained or be resolved by defense mechanisms. Sometimes the infected area may be walled off and lie dormant for long periods of time.

Specific Resistance to Infection

Specific resistance can be either innate or acquired. Innate immunity is specific, that is, certain animals are not susceptible to specific diseases contacted by other animals or humans and vice versa. Acquired immunity may be natural or artificially acquired.

Acquired natural immunity occurs with recovery from an illness. The degree of immunity produced will vary with the disease, the person's immune system and other conditions. This type of immunity may be short or long lasting.

Artificially acquired natural immunity results from the stimulation of antibodies through vaccinations (e.g. tetanus, diphtheria, small pox). This type of immunity develops about two weeks after vaccination and is usually long lasting.

Artificially acquired passive immunity results from the transfer of antibodies. Purified serum obtained from immune individuals is given by injection to the susceptible individual. This type of immunity may be used to combat diseases such as hepatitis and rabies where protection is needed immediately.

It is short lasting, usually only a few weeks, being effective only until the administered antibodies are destroyed.

That antibodies are produced in response to both lower and upper urinary tract infections under certain conditions has been demonstrated.[2-4] The role that antibody production may play in the prevention of urinary tract infection is still not clear.

The ability of the body's immune system to produce antibodies and enzymes is being used in the development of new tests designed to aid in the determination of the presence, location and invasiveness of bacteria. Antibody-coated bacteria and lactic-dehydrogenase determinations are discussed in Chapter XII, "Localization Procedures."

BACTERIAL MORPHOLOGY AND PHYSIOLOGY

Microorganisms were first reported by Robert Hooke in 1664 when he described the fruiting bodies of mold, but it was not until 1684 with the invention of the microscope by Antoni van Leuwenhoek that microorganisms were seen in some detail. In 1876 Robert Koch proposed the germ theory of illness and established the principles for attributing an illness to a specific microorganism. These principles are known as Koch's Postulates and are still applied today when establishing the etiology of a specific illness.

In the years since these early findings, with more advanced technology and research procedures, much has been learned about the microbial world. Discoveries continue at a rapid pace, challenging health care professionals to keep up with new information. The material presented here is only a brief review of the basic structures, growth requirements and reproduction of bacteria to help the reader develop a better understanding of the prevention and control of infectious diseases.

Basic Structures

Bacteria vary in size from approximately 0.5 to 6 microns (1 micron equals approximately 1/25,000 of an inch). They occur in a variety of shapes, cocci (round), rod, filament, spiral and spiral helix (Fig. III-1). Bacteria may occur singly, in pairs, chains or clusters, with each pattern being more or less characteristic of the species of bacteria. They are comprised of organic and inorganic matter. All bacteria contain some structures that are essential to their existence, such as a cell membrane and a nuclear region containing the genetic material of the cell (Fig. III-2). They may also contain some structures for specialized function such as flagella, pili, capsule, slime layer and spores.

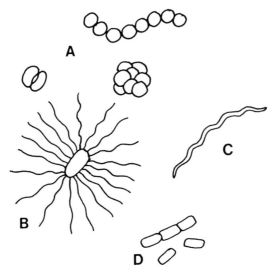

Figure III-1. Bacterial shapes and arrangements. A. Spheres (cocci), slightly elongated in pair, in chain and in cluster. B. Rod with multiple flagella. C. Spiral. D. Rods in chain and single.

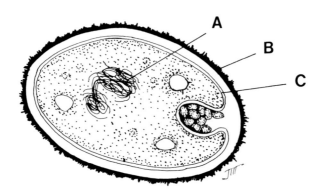

Figure III-2. Bacterial cell. A. Nuclear material. B. Cell wall. C. Cell membrane.

The *cell wall* confers rigidity and shape to the bacterium. It is permeable and allows passage of substances to and from the cell. Most bacteria can be divided into two general classifications based upon the character of their cell wall. The type of cell wall is determined through a simple staining process known as the *Gram stain,* and they are classified as either Gram-positive or Gram-negative based on the type of stain retained by the cell. The difference in affinity of stain is considered to be due to differences in composition of the cell wall. Gram-positive organisms are thought to have a thick peptidoglycan layer (e.g. staphylococcus), while Gram-negative organisms have a thinner peptidoglycan layer covered by lipopolysaccharide and protein layers (e.g. *Escherichia coli*). Knowledge of the Gram stain reaction of a specific bacteria is of value if treatment is necessary before antibiotic sensitivity results are available, as certain antibiotics are known to be more effective against either Gram-positive or Gram-negative organisms. Some disinfectants are also more effective against one type than the other.

The cells of some species of bacteria are surrounded by a *capsule* or *slime* layer which protects them from the environment and which make them more difficult to erradicate. The slime layer also enables bacteria to cling to a surface more tenaciously (e.g. *Klebsiella*).

Beneath the cell wall is a finer *cell membrane* which is a critical barrier between the cell and the environment and has pores which open and close to allow passage of material to and from the cell (Fig. III-2).

Some bacteria exhibit active motility as the result of thin appendages. The appendages are free at one end and attached to the cell at the other end. They may occur singular, in pairs, in clusters, or surround the surface of the cell. If they are long they are called *flagella* and if short, they are called *pili* (Fig. III-3). It is important to keep the motility of bacteria in mind when considering the prevention of infection, since motile bacteria will swim from one area to another if a fluid path is available (e.g. in urine drainage tubing, catheters, moist areas). Even those bacteria that have no active motility will travel from one area to another through a process called *Brownian movement*, with the bacterial cell being bombarded by elements in the environment and gradually moved from one area to another.

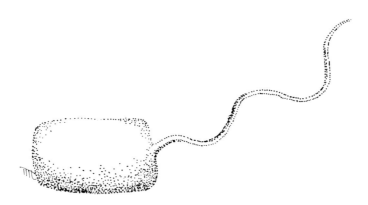

Figure III-3. Bacterial cell with flagellum.

Certain rod-shaped bacteria are able to convert themselves into a resting stage called a *spore*. The bacterial cells lose water and condense into a thick-walled round form which is capable of surviving adverse conditions that would kill the vegetative cell. When conditions are favorable, these spores will germinate into a productive cell again. Many disinfectants capable of destroying bacterial cells will be ineffective against spores so that processes, such as steam under pressure (autoclaving), may be necessary to effectively sterilize an object.

Growth Requirements

As with all living things, bacteria have certain environmental or growth requirements. *Temperature* is a critical factor and most bacteria will tolerate no more than a 10- to 20-degree temperature range. Some bacteria will grow best at high temperatures and others at low temperatures. Unfortunately, most bacteria causing urinary tract infection grow best at body temperature.

All bacteria require *oxygen* to grow. Some require free oxygen and are called *aerobes* and some obtain their oxygen chemically from material in which they are growing and are called *anaerobes.* Strict anaerobes are unable to grow when exposed to air. Still a third group of bacteria are able to adapt and use either source of oxygen. They are called *facultative.* Bacteria causing urinary tract infections are usually aerobic or facultative. However, studies have shown that anaerobes may also cause urinary tract infections.[5] This should be kept in mind if a patient demonstrates the symptoms of a urinary tract infection but has sterile urine on routine cultures. Urine for anaerobic culture must be obtained in a special manner and cultured anaerobically. At present, not all laboratories routinely perform anaerobic urine cultures.

The *nutrient* requirements will vary for different species of bacteria. The classification of bacteria is based in part on the ability of organisms to grow in specific nutrients. Some organisms are difficult to grow in the laboratory because they have complex nutritional requirements. These organisms are called *fastidious.* Urine provides all the nutrients required for bacteria producing urinary tract infections.

The acidity or alkalinity of a solution is referred to as pH. Most bacteria producing urinary tract infections will grow best in a neutral (pH of 7.0) or alkaline (pH above 7.0) medium, and growth will be retarded in an acid (pH of 5.5–4.5) medium. Therefore, keeping the urine at a pH of 5.5 or less will usually retard bacterial growth.

Water is essential for bacterial growth. Drying may not actually kill bacteria, but it will slow down their metabolism and prevent them from multiplying. Replenishing the water may return them to an active state.

Reproduction and Genetic Variations

Bacteria multiply primarily by a process of asexual division. Each bacterium contains *chromosomes.* The structural units of the chromosomes are called *genes,* with each gene controlling a specific characteristic. When the bacterial cell divides asexually, each chromosome with its individual genes duplicates itself, with the new unit going to the new cell (Fig. III-4). Most bacteria causing urinary tract infections are capable of dividing asexually every twenty to thirty minutes. Transmissible changes in the genetic characteristics occur when there is a change in the genetic structure. These changes are called *mutations.* A mutation can be produced experimentally by radiation, chemicals or other agents, or they can be produced as the result of *transduction, transformation* or *sexual recombination.*

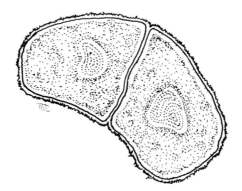

Figure III-4. Bacterial cell undergoing asexual division.

Transduction is the transfer of genetic material from one bacterial cell to another by viruses (*bacteriophages*) which live in the bacterial cell. The viruses are capable of acquiring genetic material from the host cell, leaving the host cell and entering another host cell. If the two bacterial cells have different genetic patterns and the genetic material from the virus is incorporated into the chromosomes of the new host cell, a *mutation* occurs. The new host cell will then have acquired some of the characteristics of the first cell. These characteristics will be passed on to succeeding generations through asexual reproduction.

Transformation involves a similar transfer of genetic material from one bacterial cell to another but without the intervention of a virus to "transport" the genetic material. Genetic material is released from one cell by dissolution of the cell, then absorbed by another cell which may incorporate it into its nuclear apparatus to produce new characteristics.

Sexual recombination occurs when there is a transfer of genetic material from one type of cell (male) to another (female). This probably occurs during some form of cellular conjugation. All new cells produced will have the characteristics of both parent cells.

Mutations play an important role in the ability of bacteria to produce disease and resist antibiotics.

Bacterial Variants, Protoplasts, and L-Forms

Under certain conditions, the cell wall of some bacteria will lyse or be destroyed to leave what is called a *protoplast* or *L-form*.[6] Without the rigid cell wall, they take on an irregular form but retain the ability to grow and multiply. Cell walls may lyse in the presence of those antibiotics that act by interfering with cell wall synthesis. For example, some strains of *Proteus* will produce L-forms in the presence of ampicillin. Protoplasts or L-forms are not affected by the ampicillin and have been shown to regain a cell wall when freed from exposure to the antibiotic. It has been suggested that if a patient has recurrent urinary tract infection with an organism prone to produce L-forms, treatment with an antibiotic that affects cell wall synthesis (such as ampicillin) should be followed by a course of treatment with an antibiotic having another method of activity, such as erythromycin, which acts by preventing ribosome transfer during protein synthesis.[7] L-forms have been isolated from urine, but this requires a more elaborate culture procedure and is not practical for routine cultures.[7]

Plasmids, R-factors

Plasmids are small particles within the bacterial cell containing genetic material. They are not located upon the chromosomes, but they are duplicated and transmitted to new cells during asexual cell division. Some of the plasmids may contain the genetic material that transmits to the bacterial cell its capacity to resist a given antibiotic. These plasmids are called *R-factors*. It is believed that R-factors pass from one species of organism to another through conjugation, thereby transferring antibiotic resistance to another species of organism. The antimicrobial drugs for which R-factors are able to transfer resistance include ampicillin, chloramphenicol, kanamycin, neomycin, penicillin, streptomycin, the sulfonamides and the tetracyclines.[8] This transfer of resistance factors accounts for the rapid increase in antibiotic resistance in Gram-negative organisms and is of particular concern when treating patients with long-term urinary tract problems.

BACTERIURIA—ETIOLOGY

Before discussing the individual species of bacteria, it might be well to review some of the classification criteria. Many laboratories will make a preliminary report of organisms which are present before final identification is clear. This is first based on the result of the Gram stain. The report will state Gram-positive or Gram-negative. The next classification often relates to the organism's ability to metabolize lactose and would be reported lactose-positive or lactose-negative. Further identification might include the ability to produce or not produce the enzyme *urease*. Organisms that produce urease are known as *urea splitters,* because the enzyme urease enables them to break down the urea in the urine to ammonia and carbon dioxide. The ammonia converts the urine to an alkaline medium facilitating more rapid bacterial growth. Urea splitters are often associated with urinary calculi formation.

If a laboratory sends out a preliminary report stating that the organism present was a Gram-negative, lactose-positive rod, the clinician has some idea which type of organism might be present and is better able to choose an antibiotic if treatment must be started before final identification and sensitivity patterns are available. It should be kept in mind that occasionally a variant strain of the species may develop that does not fit the general characteristics of that species challenging the microbiologists in their identification process.

Bacteria Occurring Frequently in Urine Cultures

Escherichia coli

E. coli is a Gram-negative rod. It is actively motile, urease-negative and lactose-positive. It is commonly found in the gastrointestinal tract and grows as a facultative anaerobe. *E. coli* is characterized by at least three antigenic components: flagella—H antigen, cell wall—O antigen, and capsule—K antigen. The K antigen appears to be the most important in pathogenicity.[8,9] Strains with large amounts of K antigen more commonly involve the kidney. Increased K antigen is believed to increase bacterial resistance to phagocytosis.[10] Hemolytic variants occur which produce a lysosomal enzyme which is probably also related to pathogenicity. *E. coli* is noted as the most frequent causative organism of urinary tract infections in the normal population. Its high incidence is somewhat reduced in patients with long-term urinary problems as other species increase in frequency. Some strains of *E. coli* are known to cause enteric illness.

Proteus

Proteus mirabilis and *Proteus vulgaris* are the two species now included in the genus *Proteus.* Both are actively motile Gram-negative rods. Characteristically, they produce urease which leads to alkalinization of the urine. Both species are lactose-negative. *Proteus mirabilis* is indole-negative and *Proteus vulgaris* indole-positive. Both species grow vigorously on certain culture plates. The strains which spread over the entire surface are referred to as "swarming" *Proteus. Proteus* occurs naturally in the intestinal tract of man and animals. They cause urinary tract infections and with increased frequency in patients with long-term urinary tract problems. They are frequently associated with nosocomial infections and may cause wound and burn infections, pneumonia and septicemia.[11]

Proteus morganii, formerly included in the genus *Proteus*, is now classified as *Morganella morganii.* It is a motile Gram-negative rod and it is lactose-negative. *Morganella morganii* is occasionally found in urine cultures.

Providencia

There are three species in the genus *Providencia;* they are: *P. rettgeri* (formerly called *Proteus rettgeri*), *P. stuartii*, and *P. alcalifaciens.* They are all Gram-negative motile rods, indole-positive and lactose-negative. *P. rettgeri* is urease-positive. Most strains of *Providencia* are resistant to many antibiotics. They may be found in the intestinal tract and have been the cause of hospital-associated infections, particularly in the urinary tract, wounds and burns.

Klebsiella

The species of *Klebsiella* most frequently encountered in urinary tract infection is *K. pneumoniae.* We have on rare occasions encountered *K. oxytoca* in our population of patients. Both are Gram-negative rods, non-motile and usually encapsulated. They are facultative anaerobes normally present in the intestinal tract. Their slimy capsule enables them to cling to surfaces. *K. pneumoniae* is frequently the cause of nosocomial infections, urinary tract infections, and pneumonia.

Citrobacter

Two species of *Citrobacter*, *C. freundii* and *C. diversus*, are frequently found in urine cultures of patients with long-term urinary problems. They are Gram-negative motile rods occurring normally in the intestinal tract.

Serratia

Species of *Serratia* were once regarded as harmless. Some strains, because they produce a red pigmentation, were used as test organisms to determine the effectiveness of cleaning and disinfecting procedures. *Serratia* has since been implicated as the etiological agent of many infections, particularly hospital-associated infections. *Serratia marsescens* is the species most frequently isolated from urine specimens. It is frequently resistant to many antibiotics, including aminoglycosides. It is a Gram-negative motile rod and is normally found in soil and water.

Enterobacter

Two species of the genus *Enterobacter* which we have encountered in urine cultures are *E. cloaca* and *E. sakozakii.* They are Gram-negative rods which normally may be found in the intestinal tract of man and animals. They may also be found in soil, water and dairy products. They are closely related to *Klebsiella* and some laboratories do not separate these species in reporting. Many strains of *Enterobacter* are motile.

Pseudomonas

There are several species of *Pseudomonas* associated with urinary tract infections. *Pseudomonas* usually inhabit fresh water and soil and are not generally found in the intestinal tract of humans. Although they grow easily on simple media, multiple tests are often required for identification. They are Gram-negative rods. Most species are strict aerobes.

Pseudomonas aeruginosa is a common contaminant of the hospital environment. It has been recovered from water faucets, thermometers, floors, bathrooms, showers, etc. In culture, it may produce pyocyanin, a blue pigment. Some strains produce brown or black pigments. Healthy humans are usually not infected by *Pseudomonas aeruginosa.* However, they occur frequently in blood, urine and exudate from patients with reduced natural resistance. It is found with relatively high frequency in urine from patients using long-term urinary drainage appliances. It has been found as a contaminant in various soaps and disinfection agents. It is frequently resistant to many antibiotics.

Pseudomonas pseudomallei is commonly found in moist soil in Southeast Asia and North Australia. In man, it can cause *Melioidosis,* which is a disease that may be characterized by toxic pneumonia and overwhelming septicemia. It was a concern during the Vietnam War.[8] We have found it occasionally in urine specimens from our patients.

Pseudomonas maltophilia is an organism that causes the disease *Glanders* in horses and can be transmitted to humans, where it may cause respiratory tract infections.[8] We have on rare occasions found it in urine cultures. *P. maltophilia* is often quite resistant to antibiotics. It is a non-motile Gram-negative rod.

Pseudomonas cepacia is another species of Pseudomonas found on very rare occasions in the urine. It is more commonly associated with endocarditis among intravenous illicit drug users.

Streptococcus

Streptococci are round in shape. They are Gram-positive, non-motile and do not form spores. They characteristically grow in chains. When grown on sheep blood agar, they exhibit different types of hemolysis: alpha, in which the red blood cells are changed to an olive green color; beta, in which the red cells are completely lysed to form a clear pinkish zone on the agar; and gamma, where there is no hemolysis. These reactions are used to help classify *Streptococcus.* They are further classified by growth requirements and the Lancefield grouping sera. We will discuss only two of these groups, the *pyogenic group* and the *enterococcus group*, as they are the ones more frequently encountered in urine cultures.

Included in the pyogenic group are the Lancefield group B beta hemolytic *Streptococcus.* They are occasionally found in urine cultures and generally respond well to treatment with penicillin. Beta Streptococci is probably best known for its role as the causative organism of scarlet fever and rheumatic fever.

The second group of streptococcus consists of the *enterococcus.* They play a more important role in urinary tract infections. They type out as group D with the Lancefield typing sera. They are Gram-positive cocci occurring normally in the intestinal tract. Although they are found quite frequently in urine cultures, they tend to remain in the lower urinary tract and seldom produce pyelonephritis.

Staphylococcus

Staphylococcus are Gram-positive non-motile, non-spore-forming cocci. Some strains are encapsulated. They grow singly, in pairs or in clusters. There are two species that occasionally occur in urine cultures: *Staphylococcus aureus* and *Staphylococcus epidermidis. Staphylococcus aureus* is hemolytic, lysing red blood cells in culture media. Some strains of *Staphylococcus aureus* produce an enzyme called *coagulase.* It is believed that organisms that are coagulase-positive are more pathogenic. Therefore, many laboratories will report the coagulase reaction. *Staphylococcus epidermidis* is present on human skin. *Staphylococcus aureus* may also be present on the skin of some individuals from which they can be transferred to other susceptible individuals. *Staphylococcus aureus* is more frequently implicated in food poisoning, wound infections, and skin infections, including impetigo, than in urinary tract infections. *Staphylococcus epidermidis* seems to be a less pathogenic organism but has been reported to cause urinary tract infections.[12]

Other microorganisms occurring with less frequency in urinary cultures

Acinetobacter is a Gram-negative rod. It is non-motile, non-fermentative, and aerobic, formerly classified under the genus *Neisseria*. It is oxidase negative and penicillin resistant and is readily isolated from soil and water.

Eckenella corroden is a Gram-negative rod occasionally isolated from the respiratory tract. Literature indicates it is sensitive to ampicillin, penicillin, carbenicillin, and tetracycline. Although we have found it in urine cultures, the pathogenicity of this organism is questionable.

Borditella bronchisepticia is small Gram-negative, motile coccobacillus (very short small rods resembling cocci). It is a rapid urea splitter. It is found in animals and can cause bronchopneumonia in pigs and rabbits. In humans, it occasionally produces a pertussis-like disease. We have found it in urine cultures.

Candida albicans is a yeast frequently present in the alimentary tract and vagina. In urine cultures it is often associated with long-term antibiotic treatment. *Candida* will occasionally produce a symptomatic urinary tract infection.[13]

BACTERIURIA—URINARY TRACT INFECTION

How is knowledge of bacteria and the infection process related to long-term urinary tract care? How and where do bacteria gain entry into the urinary tract, and when and where do they cause problems?

Bacteria may reach the urinary tract from sites within the body through the lymphatic or circulatory system, but the most common source is believed to be from outside the body. We know that bacteria can migrate, so they can travel from outside the body ascending into the urethra and eventually into the bladder. Cleanliness of the perineal area will reduce the number of potential pathogens. *Escherichia coli* is an organism found most frequently in urine cultures of persons having normally functioning urinary tracts, probably because it is actively motile. Existing in large numbers in the gastrointestinal tract, it migrates from there to the urinary tract through moisture in the perineal area. *E. coli* has a rapid growth rate and will often overgrow other types of bacteria which are present. However, as we shall see later, people with neurogenic bladders with or without urinary drainage appliances often have other bacteria occurring more frequently than *E. coli.*

Maintaining the integrity of the urethral mucosa will prevent many bacteria from penetrating the cells where they can grow and multiply. Consequently, invasive procedures should be conducted with care.

Insufficiently lubricated catheters can irritate the mucosa during passage through the urethra. Excessive force in passing the catheter past an obstructed sphincter or stricture may also produce tissue damage and lead to development of a urethral diverticulum (false passage). If a diverticulum develops, urine will pool, become stagnant and allow bacteria to grow. If an infection develops in the urethra, it is called *urethritis.* As the body's defense mechanisms go to work, inflammation develops which results in swelling, making passage of a catheter even more difficult. In the presence of an indwelling catheter, purulent exudates can collect on the catheter, forming crusty accumulations which may further irritate the meatus and urethra, perpetuate infection and provide a pathway for bacterial migration.

If the bacteria gain access to the bladder, *bacteriuria* occurs. The normal bladder has several natural defense mechanisms to prevent bacteriuria from resulting in infection. The first mechanism is the antibacterial properties of urine itself due to its normally acid pH. The second mechanism is the washing action of the urine flow. Consistently adequate fluid intake and frequent bladder emptying will reduce the bacterial count in the urine. Thirdly, there is evidence that phagocytosis may occur on the surface of the bladder mucosa.[7] Fourthly, the mucopolysaccharide on the surface of the bladder epithelium is believed to act as an anti-adherence factor to prevent bacteria from adhering to the bladder surface. Other antibacterial defense mechanisms are believed to exist but have not yet been defined. If the bladder defenses are not sufficient to prevent the bacteria from becoming established in the tissues, infection (*cystitis*) develops.

In an abnormal bladder (neurogenic or with other pathology), such normal defense mechanisms may be ineffective. Bladder diverticula or trabeculations will permit the urine to pool and become stagnant, preventing effective bladder washouts. Large residuals remaining after incomplete bladder emptying will also prevent bladder "washout" and promote stagnation of the urine. Irritation of the bladder endothelium by foreign objects (catheter or bladder calculi) will provide a place for bacteria to penetrate the tissue, grow and spread. Overdistention due to bladder outlet obstruction, plugged or kinked catheters or tubing, full collecting device or sphincter dyssynergia can result in damage to the bladder mucosa and often results in cystitis. It is believed that the neurogenic bladder mucosa also loses some of its normal antibacterial activity.[14]

As the body responds to infection, inflammation of the bladder wall occurs causing swelling and irritation. The urine becomes cloudy and bleeding may occur, resulting in *hematuria*. Bladder infections may be acute, responding to effective treatment, or may become chronic with the development of hypertrophy and scarring, resulting in poor bladder wall contractability and the perpetuation of infection.

If bacteria ascend into the ureter, infection may occur (e.g. *ureteritis*). Certain bacteria are known to produce toxins (e.g. *E. coli*) that paralyze the muscles in the ureteral walls, prohibiting the normal peristaltic activity.[15] Urine then progresses from the kidneys to the bladder both by the force of gravity and pressure from newly formed urine emerging from the kidneys. If infection persists, the ureters may become stretched, distended and tortuous.

Although lower urinary tract infections may be severe and painful, of even greater importance is infection within the kidney itself (*pyelonephritis*). Bacterial pyelonephritis may be acute or chronic. A single acute infection if promptly treated will usually result in little loss of renal function. However, repeated acute infections or a continual chronic infection can lead to severe loss of renal function (Fig. III-5). Bacteria may penetrate and grow in one of several localized areas within the kidney producing abscesses. Promptly treated, the infection is usually cleared and replaced by scar tissue. However, at times the areas become walled off remaining dormant for varying periods, later releasing bacteria and thus perpetuating the infection. For this reason, persons with urinary tract abnormalities such as a neurogenic bladder should have periodic evaluations to determine if chronic infection is resulting in scarring and in decreased renal function.

The diagnosis of a urinary tract infection is based at least in part on the urine culture result. Methods for obtaining cultures and interpreting results are discussed in Chapter XII.

The presence of bacteria is readily established by culture procedures, but determining the significance of bacteriuria is more difficult. In 1956, Kass[16] reported on the use of a colony count to differentiate significant from non-significant bacteriuria, with colony counts of 100,000 col/ml or greater considered significant. This criterion can still be used with some validity, especially in screening tests conducted on given populations using clean catch urine specimens. However, for persons with long-term urinary problems, a significant colony count may be considerably lower. For instance, because of the smaller volume of the ileal conduit, Spence and co-workers[17] found that colony counts of 10,000 col/ml in a specimen taken from the conduit were significant.

It has been shown that in other persons with chronic pyelonephritis, the colony counts may be less than 10,000 col/ml, as only a few bacteria may escape to appear in the urine at one time.[18,19]

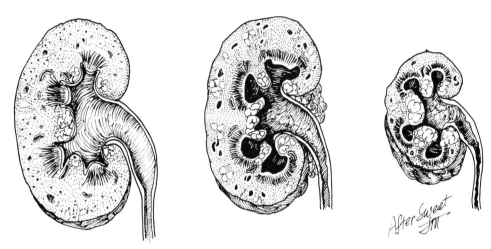

Figure III-5. Chronic pyelonephritis. Progression of scarring and diminution of renal parenchyma.

It is our belief that colony counts of less than 100,000 col/ml often are significant not only for patients with ileal diversion but for many other patients, including those with long-term urinary problems. We, with others, have found that if two successive cultures exhibit the same organism, even in small concentrations, it is an indication of existing infection. Unfortunately, many patients who have long-term urinary tract problems have additional disabilities that make it physically difficult and financially burdensome to seek medical care. Therefore, one culture result is often all that is obtainable and treatment must be based on that result.

Likewise, symptomatology is not always of assistance to the clinician, since many patients, such as the spinal cord injured, will not demonstrate the classic symptoms of a urinary tract infection. Symptoms they may experience are increased spasticity, headaches, cloudy, foul smelling or bloody urine. Some will experience fever and chills. Fever, at least in the spinal cord injured, can be relative because these patients normally often have lower temperatures than 98.6° F. It is not unusual for them to have temperatures as low as 96° F. Presenting with a temperature of 99° F would then indicate a 3° fever. It is necessary to inquire as to the patient's normal temperature.

All of these things do indeed challenge the clinician responsible for the patient's care. Other tests to help evaluate significance of bacteriuria are discussed in Chapter XII.

E.N.

REFERENCES

1. Wilson, M.E., and Mizer, H.E.: *Microbiology and Patient Care*, 2nd ed. New York, MacMillan, 1974.
2. Hand, W.L., Smith, J.W., Miller, T.E., Barnett, J.A. and Sanford, J.P.: Immunoglobulin synthesis in lower urinary tract infection. *J Lab and Clin Med 75*:19–29, 1970.
3. Whitworth, J.A., Fairley, K., O'Keefe, C.M. and Miller, T.E.: Immunogenicity of *Eschiricia coli* antigen in upper urinary tract infection. *Kidney Int 8*:316–319, 1975.
4. Jodal, U., Ahlstedt, S., Carlsson. B., Hanson, L.A., Lindberg, U., and Sohl, A.: Local antibodies in childhood urinary tract infection. A Preliminary Study. *Int Arch Allergy 47*:537–546, 1974.
5. Ribot, S., Gal, K., Goldblat, M.V., and Eslami, H.H.: The role of anaerobic bacteria in the pathogenesis of urinary tract infections. *J Urol 126*:852–853, 1981.
6. Guinan, P.D., Neter, E., and Murphy, G.P.: The significance of L-forms in human renal disease. *J Urol 108*:50–53, 1972.
7. Kunin, C.M.: *Detection, Prevention and Management of Urinary Tract Infections.* 3rd ed. Philadelphia, Lea and Febiger, 1979.
8. Milgrom, F., and Flanagan, T.D. (Eds.): *Medical Microbiology.* New York, Churchill Livingstone, 1982.
9. Bailey, W.R., and Scott, E.G.: *Diagnostic Microbiology.* 3rd ed. St. Louis, C.V. Mosby, 1970.
10. Glynn, A.A., Brumfitt, W., and Howard, C.J.: K antigens of *Eschirichia coli* and renal involvement in urinary tract infections. *Lancet 1*:514–516, 1971.
11. Washington, J.A., Senjem, D.H., Haldorson, A., Schutt, A.H., and Martin, W.J.: Nosocomially acquired bacteriuria due to *Proteus rettgeri* and *Providencia stuartii. Amer J Clin Path 60*:836–838, 1973.
12. Bailey, R.R.: Significance of coagulase negative *Staphylococcus* in urine. *J Infect Disease 127*:179–182, 1973.
13. Zincke, H., Furlow, W.L., and Farrow, G.M.: *Candida albicans* cystitis. Report of a case with special emphasis on diagnosis and treatment. *J Urol 109*:612–614, 1973.
14. Perez, J.R., Grieco, E.R., and Gillenwater, J.Y.: Evidence for bladder bactericidal factor. *Invest Urol 11*:489–495, 1974.
15. Boyarsky, S., and Lebay, P.C.: *Ureteral Dynamics, Pathophysiology, Drugs and Surgical Implications.* Baltimore, Williams and Wilkins Co., 1972.
16. Kass, E.H.: Asymptomatic infections of the urinary tract. *Trans Assoc of Am Physicians 69*:56–64, 1956.
17. Spence, B., Stewart, W., and Cass, A.S.: Use of a double lumen catheter to determine bacteriuria in intestinal loop diversion in children. *J Urol 108*:800, 1972.
18. Stamey, T.A.: *Pathogenesis and Treatment of Urinary Tract Infections.* Baltimore/London, Williams and Wilkins, 1980.
19. Effersøe, P., and Jensen, E.: Urinary tract infection versus bacterial contamination; A quantitative study. *Lancet 1*:1342–1343, 1963.

Chapter IV

METHODS OF URINARY DRAINAGE

The urine formed by the kidneys must be eliminated from the body if good urinary tract function is to be maintained. Normally, this is achieved through the process of micturition. Injury, aging or disease may temporarily or permanently affect the normal process, and incontinence, hesitancy, frequency or the inability to void may result.

Through the years several methods of urinary drainage have been devised to help alleviate these problems. The most common methods are indwelling urethral or suprapubic catheters, external catheters, supravesical diversion and intermittent catheterization. Each method will be discussed in detail in succeeding chapters.

Indwelling catheters are, as the name implies, catheters that are inserted into the bladder to continuously drain the urine. These catheters are so constructed that they are retained within the bladder for periods of time. The most common method of insertion of the catheter into the bladder is through the urethra. This is called *indwelling urethral catheterization* but is commonly referred to as simply *indwelling* catheterization (see Chap. V).

A second method of insertion is through a surgical incision in the abdominal and bladder walls. This is called *indwelling suprapubic catheterization* and is usually referred to simply as *suprapubic catheterization* (Chap. VI).

Male patients may be maintained with an *external catheter.* An external catheter is an appliance which is attached to or surrounds the penis in such a manner that urine is collected as it is expelled and is drained away from the penis into a urine collecting appliance. External catheters are discussed in Chapter VII.

The *appliance-free state* implies the natural method of bladder filling and emptying. However, patients with neurogenic bladders may require physiological and pharmacological management and close follow-up to safely maintain an appliance-free state (see Chapter IX).

An *intermittent catheterization* program may be used by some patients. The bladder is emptied periodically by inserting a catheter through the urethra into the bladder to drain the urine. This procedure is discussed in Chapter VIII.

Supravesical urinary diversion is a method of urinary drainage in which a surgical procedure bypasses the urinary bladder. We will be discussing in Chapter X the ileal and sigmoid conduit types of urinary diversions. These types of drainage involve the construction of an "artificial" bladder or conduit from a segment of the ileum or colon into which the ureters drain. Urine then empties from the conduit through an opening in the abdominal wall into an appliance which is attached to the outside of the body.

The maintenance of good urinary tract function while using any of these methods of drainage is dependent upon the prevention of damage to the urinary tract due to infection or conditions such as overdistention, reflux and calculi.

COMMON POTENTIAL DANGERS

Potential dangers common to all types of urinary drainage are infection, calculi and tissue damage. They will be discussed briefly here and then referred to in succeeding chapters with the conditions or problems that are specific for each method of drainage.

Infection

The incidence of bacteriuria in persons using any type of urinary drainage appliance is high and the patterns of organism isolation and symptoms of infection are frequently different from those encountered in the general population. This is discussed in Chapter XI. Infection, bacteriuria and urinary tract infections have been discussed in detail in Chapter III.

In review, urinary tract infections refer to infections of the urinary tract which may be symptomatic or asymptomatic regardless of location in the bladder, ureter or kidneys.

Bladder infection (cystitis), though of concern itself, can lead to even more severe urinary tract problems. Recurrent or chronic cystitis may result in the development of reflux because the anti-reflux mechanism becomes swollen and inefficient. The reflux of urine through the ureter may result in ureteritis and/or pyelonephritis and ultimately diminished kidney function.

An episode of acute pyelonephritis, if promptly and successfully treated, will produce some scarring in the kidneys but generally will not severely affect kidney function. However, repeated episodes of pyelonephritis will lead to massive scarring of the renal tissue, the development of calyceal blunting and eventually diminished kidney function.

Calculi

Calculi (stones) form as a result of the crystalization of mineral salts. In humans, urinary tract stones are usually formed from calcium oxalate, calcium phosphate, uric acid, magnesium ammonium phosphate or cystine.[1] Before a stone can form, the urine must be supersaturated. That is, it must contain more of a substance than can be held in solution permanently.

When conditions are favorable the mineral salts in the supersaturated urine are deposited upon a nucleus or nidus, which may be any particle or debris and is frequently bacteria. Crystals are deposited upon the nidus in layers. Often, layers of bacteria are dispersed between layers of crystals.[1]

The risk of calculi in immobilized patients and patients with long-term urinary tract problems is high, particularly in those patients with untreated urinary tract infections.[1] When stones occur, a comprehensive work-up is needed to identify the type of stones present and to establish a care program.

Several conditions including low fluid intake, stasis, infection, immobilization, hypercalciuria, urinary pH, and a prior history of stone disease increase the risk of stone formation. Good management can do much to minimize these risks.

Low Fluid Intake

A fluid intake sufficient to produce an urinary output of at least 2,000 ml per day will usually maintain the urine in an unsaturated state. Frequent monitoring of fluid output will help to appraise intake and encourage patient compliance. There should be sufficient fluid intake evenings and at night, as well as at regular intervals during the day, to insure that the urine is unsaturated at all times.[2]

Stasis

Stasis, the stoppage of the flow or discharge of urine, may occur at any level of the urinary tract. When stasis occurs there is a greater period of time during which the urine may be in contact with a nidus. If the urine is supersaturated, there is more opportunity for crystalization of minerals onto the nidus. Frequent turning or changing the position of a patient will help to "empty out" stagnant urine from places where it is collecting, for instance, from saccules, diverticula or below the tip of the catheter. See Chapter XVII "Urinary Calculi" for additional information regarding urinary calculi.

Infection

Infection is perhaps the greatest contributing factor to stone disease. Consistent monitoring and prompt treatment of infection will do much to minimize the risk of stone formation.

Microorganisms that produce the enzyme urease are called "urea splitters." Some commonly occurring urea splitters are species of *Proteus, Providencia,* and *Enterobacter.* They are important bacteria contributing to stone formation because they break down urea present in the urine to form ammonia which alkalinizes the urine. Stones such as magnesium-ammonium phosphate and calcium-phosphate-carbonate form more readily in supersaturated urine that is alkaline.

Bacteria also play another role in stone formation, as they can form the nucleus upon which crystals are deposited. Once stones are present, infections are very difficult to clear up because the bacteria become incorporated into the stone and cling to the surface.[3]

Immobilization Hypercalciuria

When there is a decrease in stress to bones with immobilization there is a loss of bone material to the blood which can result in hypercalciuria and a supersaturation of the urine with calcium oxalate or calcium phosphate. Studies have shown that gravitational stress on bones produced by standing for two hours daily will decrease the loss of calcium from the bones and decrease urinary calcium.[4,5] More studies are necessary to determine whether standing for frequent shorter intervals will have the same effect.

Urinary pH

It is usually desirable to maintain an acid urine. An acid urine tends to increase the solubility of potential stone-forming minerals, thereby decreasing the risk of calculi such as calcium-oxalate and calcium-phosphate. An alkaline pH, which is frequently produced if urea-splitting organisms are present, will increase the danger of formation of these types of stones. On the other hand, uric acid stones tend to form more readily in an acid urine. Alkalinization of the urine may be desirable for patients who tend to form uric acid stones. Knowledge of the types of stones produced by the patient will aid in management.

Mechanical Damage

Care must be taken to use proper procedures for the placement and handling of urinary drainage appliances to prevent damage to the urinary tract tissue. Tissue damage may result from poor catheterization procedures, improper placement of external catheter or ostomy appliances, as well as the improper placement and handling of drainage tubing and urine collection receptacles. These dangers will be further discussed with reference to each method of drainage and in Chapter XI.

E.N.

REFERENCES

1. Resnick, M.I., and Boyce, W.H.: Aetiological theories of renal lithiasis—a historical review. In Wickham, J.E.A. (Ed.): *Urinary Calculus Disease.* Edinburgh, London and New York, Churchill Livingstone, 1979, pp. 1–20.
2. Thomas, W.C., Jr.: Medical aspects of renal calculus disease. *Urologic Clinics of North Am* 1:261–278, 1974.
3. Nemoy, N.J., and Stamey, T.A.: Surgical, bacteriological and biochemical management of "infection stones". *JAMA 215:*1470–1476, 1971.
4. Smith, P.H., and Robertson, W.G.: Stone formation in the immobilized patient. In Hodgkins, A., and Nordin, B.E.C.: *Renal Stone Research Symposium.* London, Churchill, 85–92.
5. Donaldson, C.L., Hulley, S.B., Vogel, J.M., Hattner, R.S., Bayers, J.H., and McMillan, D.E.: Effect of prolonged bedrest on bone mineral. *Metabolism 19:*1071–1084, 1970.

Chapter V

INDWELLING URETHRAL CATHETERS

U rine retention has probably occurred since early mankind. Ancient writings suggest that methods were found to drain the bladder as far back as 3000 B.C. In later years, the Chinese, Egyptians, Greeks and Romans are known to have devised ingenious methods to empty a distended bladder. Early "catheters" were apparently metal tubes that were inserted into the bladder through the urethra. The Arabians are credited with developing a flexible catheter in the eleventh century. During the eighteenth century catheters were devised of silver and woven silk. In the early 1900s and up to about 1930, all woven catheters used in the United States were manufactured in Europe, particularly France and Germany. Because of fear that in the event of war catheters might not be available from other sources, an effort was made to develop and manufacture catheters in the United States, and in 1939 the first American made catheters were available. Instead of woven silk, woven nylon was used which was coated with a synthetic resin coating.[1] Since that time, great improvements have been made in both the materials used and the size and shape that eventually lead to the development of catheters as we know them today.

INDICATIONS FOR USE

The most common indications for use of a long-term indwelling urethral catheter are incontinence or the inability to void. They may also be used for convenience or to help a patient gain more independence.

Incontinence in a male is managed with an external catheter when possible, but some patients find it difficult to keep an external catheter in place or develop excoriations on the shaft of the penis, necessitating an indwelling catheter. To date, there are no satisfactory external catheters for females; so, if padding and protective clothing do not meet the patient's needs, an indwelling catheter may be used.

If bladder emptying cannot be accomplished by triggered, spontaneous or at-will voiding, either an indwelling catheter or intermittent catheterization will be necessary to prevent bladder overdistention, unless there is surgical intervention such as a sphincterotomy.

71

An indwelling catheter is occasionally used as a matter of convenience and for independence—for example, for patients whose daily activities require them to be in locations where facilities are not available for intermittent catheterization or a triggered voiding program, or who do not have the assistance necessary for that type of management. However, the inherent dangers of an indwelling catheter must be carefully measured against the value of convenience and independence.

INHERENT DANGERS

There are three major factors contributing to the inherent danger of an indwelling catheter. These are infection, calculi and mechanical tissue damage.

Infection

Bacteriuria is a common occurrence with long-term indwelling catheters. In fact, it has been shown that bacteriuria will usually occur within two weeks after a catheter is in place.[2] It is important, then, to prevent the bacteria present in the urine from causing damage. This can best be done by keeping the concentration of organisms present in the urine low to minimize the effects of toxins produced by the bacteria and by preventing damage to urinary tract tissue so that bacteria cannot penetrate the tissue and produce an "infection."

The role of fluid intake, diet and urine acidification in the prevention and control of infection will be discussed later in this chapter. The organism isolation patterns for patients with indwelling urethral catheters will be discussed in Chapter XI.

Danger Areas

Three main danger areas where bacteria may enter the system are: the perineal area, catheter-tubing junction, and the tubing and collecting appliance (Fig. V-1).

Perineal Area: During the initial catheterization, care must be taken to prevent contamination from the environment or by insertion of the catheter through an improperly prepared site.

Bacteria can migrate from the outside into the bladder between the catheter and the urethral mucosa.[3] Therefore, the meatus, perineal area and exposed portion of the catheter should be cleaned twice daily with a povidone-iodine solution (or soap and water) to minimize the number of bacteria in the area (Fig. V-1). Crustations should be removed from the meatal area and the catheter, as this material forms an excellent place for bacteria to flourish.

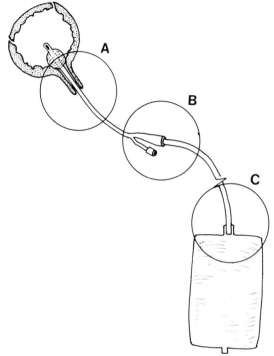

Figure V-1. Danger areas where bacteria can enter the system. A. Perineal area. B. Catheter-tubing junction. C. Tubing and urine collecting appliance.

If an erection occurs in a male, this material may be drawn up into the urethra, where it can scratch and irritate. Remember, that any time there is an irritation or breakdown of tissue, there is a place where bacteria may grow, multiply and spread into the surrounding tissue or to the bloodstream.

A recent study suggests that meatal care is not necessary and, in fact, may do more harm than good.[4] However, this study was conducted in an acute care facility on patients with short-term indwelling catheters and does not apply to long-term catheterization. Gentle, but thorough cleansing of the meatus, perineal area and the exposed length of catheter is necessary to minimize the number of bacteria that can gain access to the bladder through the meatus.

Catheter-Tubing Union: The catheter-tubing union is a frequent source of bacterial contamination (Fig. V-1). The culture plates pictured in Figure V-2 show bacterial growth in cultures made from a sterile swab that was wiped over the end of the catheter at the catheter-tubing junction before and after vigorous rubbing with alcohol.

The fingertips and fingernails should not come into direct contact with the catheter and tubing during separation. Never roll back the catheter with

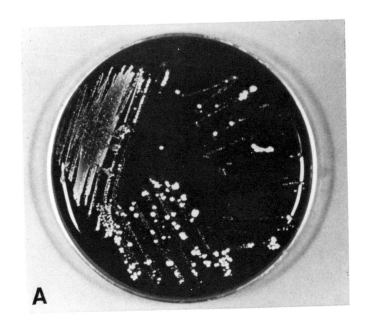

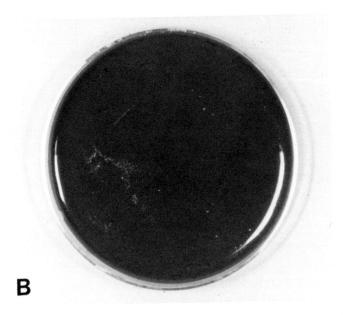

Figure V-2 A–B. Culture plates inoculated with sterile swabs that had been wiped around the end of the catheter at the catheter-tubing junction. A. Before wiping the area with 70 percent alcohol. B. After vigorously wiping the area with 70 percent alcohol.

fingertips to remove it from the tubing, as this will permit transfer of bacteria from the fingertips to the inside of the catheter (Fig. V-3).

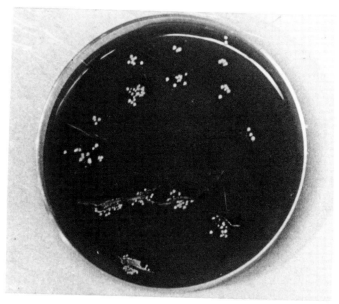

Figure V-3. Culture plate showing bacterial growth from fingertips and fingernails.

Vigorously wipe the catheter-tubing union with alcohol wipes or povidone-iodine wipes and then hold the catheter and tubing with the wipes while separating them (Fig. V-4). The open ends of the catheter and tubing should always be covered with alcohol wipes or sterile gauze pads until reconnected.

It is sometimes very difficult to connect the catheter and tubing, because they are close to the same size. This problem can be solved by using a tubing with a tapered end or one of several types of connectors (Fig. V-5).

Tubing and Urine Collecting Device: The third danger area is the tubing and urine collecting device (Fig. V-1). The importance of daily disinfection and frequent replacement of equipment will be discussed later. The leg bag or night bag must always be kept below the level of the bladder, with the tubing in a straight descending position (Figs. V-6 & V-7) When transferring the collecting device from one area to another, the tubing should be clamped or pinched close to the catheter to prevent urine from flowing back into the catheter and bladder. See Chapter XI "Positioning Urinary Drainage Equipment" for complete instruction on positioning and care of appliances.

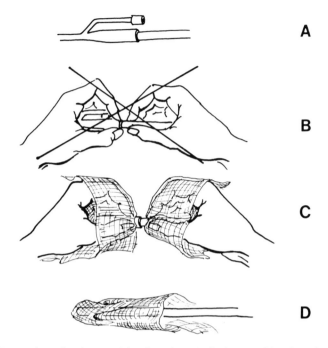

Figure V-4. Separation of catheter tubing junction. A. Catheter tubing junction. B. Improper use of fingernails and fingertips. C. Correct method after wiping with alcohol, hold tubing and catheter with sterile gauze squares. D. Cover open end of tubing or catheter with sterile gauze squares.

Calculi

Patients with long-term indwelling catheters are at risk to develop bladder or renal calculi. Approximately one-third of a population of patients with spinal cord lesions using indwelling catheters have been shown to develop bladder or renal stones.[5] Conditions favorable to the development of calculi are discussed in Chapters IV and XVII. Special emphasis should be placed on several factors for patients with indwelling catheters.

Calculi form when minerals crystalize out of a supersaturated urine onto a nidus. The high incidence of bacteriuria in this group of patients provides an ever-ready nidus. In addition, the catheter itself can serve as a nidus with minerals crystalizing onto the surface forming a layer of shale. As this shale sloughs off, it forms a nucleus upon which more crystals are deposited. It is, therefore, recommended that catheters be changed at least once a month to decrease the chance of crystalization upon the catheter surface.[6]

Stasis or pooling of urine is another problem for this group of patients, as urine tends to pool in the neck of the bladder below the catheter tip and

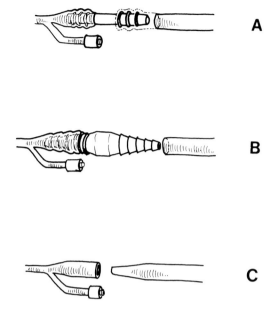

Figure V-5. Tubing connectors for indwelling catheters. A. Plastic straight connector. B. Christmas tree connector (5-in-1). C. Tapered tubing—no connector necessary.

balloon (Fig. V-8), as well as in bladder trabeculations or diverticula, providing ideal conditions for calculi to form in a bacteriuric supersaturated urine. Frequent position change will help "empty out" these pockets of stagnant urine, and good consistent fluid intake will help to dilute the urine and prevent supersaturation (Fig. V-8).

In addition to sufficient fluid intake and position change, urine acidification will help to minimize crystalization of some types of minerals.

For additional information regarding urinary calculi, see Chapter XVII, "Urinary Calculi."

Mechanical Damage

Mechanical damage to the urethra may result at the time of initial catheterization or catheter change if there is inadequate lubrication of the catheter. Approximately three inches of the tip of the catheter should be well lubricated for a female and seven inches for a male (see "Catheterization Procedures" in this chapter).

Care must be taken not to use undue force when inserting the catheter, as this could result in a false passage or development of a urethral diverticulum. If resistance is met, wait for the sphincter to relax. This may take five minutes or longer (see "Care Procedures").

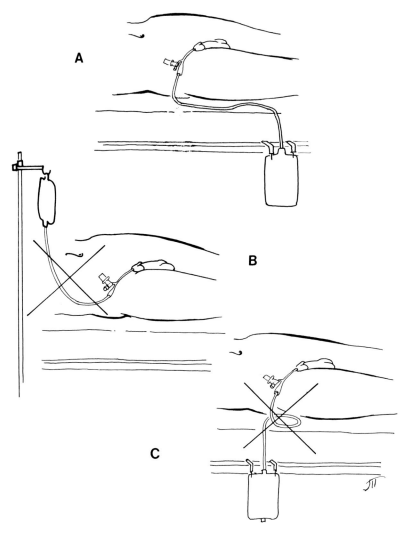

Figure V-6. Positioning indwelling catheter drainage equipment. A. Correct positioning. B. Incorrect positioning. Tubing and bag above the level of bladder. C. Incorrect positioning loop in tubing.

Tissue damage can occur in the bladder neck, urethra and meatal area from inadvertent tugging or pulling on the catheter. Anchoring the catheter to the abdomen or thigh will minimize this danger (see "Care Procedures").

Overdistention of the bladder may result from a plugged or kinked catheter or tubing or from a full collecting appliance. This overdistention may lead to the development of saccules or diverticula and result in reflux of urine through the ureters toward the kidneys. Acute overdistention can

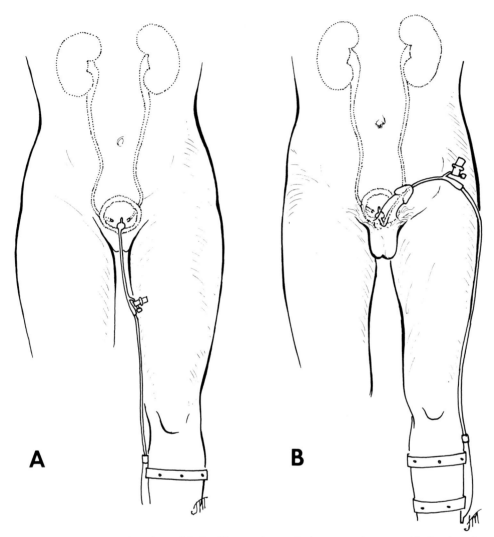

Figure V-7 A–B. Positioning of indwelling catheter drainage equipment with leg bag in proper location below the knee. A. Female. B. Male.

also lead to septicemia if bacteria gain entrance into the bloodstream through damaged blood vessels.

The bladder may also become irritated by crystals, shale or calculi as they move around within the bladder. This irritation can produce hematuria.

Remember, that any time there is irritation or damage to the tissue there is a site for bacteria to become established and cause an infection.

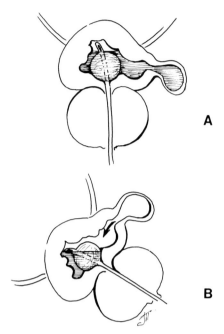

Figure V-8. Urine pooling in the bladder. A. Urine pooling below the tip of the catheter and in a bladder diverticulum. B. Urine emptying out of diverticulum with position change.

Bladder Cancer

Patients using long-term indwelling urethral catheters are at risk to develop cancer of the bladder. Studies have demonstrated that the incidence of squamous metaplasia increases with the length of time an indwelling catheter has been in use. There is a significantly greater incidence in patients who have used indwelling catheters for ten years or more.[7] Squamous metaplasia often precedes carcinoma.

The fact that squamous cell carcinoma of the bladder is considered a highly malignant neoplasm[8] further emphasizes the need for periodic comprehensive urologic evaluations for patients using indwelling catheters, including roentgenographic studies, cystoscopy and random bladder wall biopsy.[9]

EFFECT OF DIET AND FLUID INTAKE

Most bacteria causing urinary tract infections multiply by cell division with a "doubling time" of 20 to 30 minutes (see Chapter III, "Reproduction and Genetic Variations"). Good consistent fluid intake will greatly help in "washing out" bacteria before they can attain large numbers. Unless contraindicated for other medical reasons, a fluid intake adequate to insure an output of 2,000 to 3,000 ml per day is recommended, with special emphasis on an even distribution of this intake throughout the day and night.

Generally, it is best to encourage patients with indwelling catheters to drink water or cranberry juice, particularly if they are having problems with infection.

Most bacteria causing urinary tract infections grow best in a neutral or alkaline medium, while an acid urine will generally slow down or minimize bacterial growth. Medications such as ascorbic acid or ammonium chloride are sometimes given to help acidify the urine. If ammonium chloride is used, serum levels of bicarbonate should be taken to establish the correct dosage and at periodic intervals thereafter to check for possible development of acidosis.

Foods consumed will affect the pH of the urine by making the urine alkaline. The worst offenders are the citrus foods, oranges, lemons, tomatoes, etc. This may seem contradictory, since ascorbic acid (vitamin C) is sometimes given as a urine acidifier.[10] Although citrus fruits are rich in vitamin C, other substances present in these foods, such as citric acid, are metabolized to an alkaline ash and offset any acidifying effect of the vitamin C present.

This is perhaps a good time to discuss the merits of cranberry juice. Raw cranberries themselves are fairly rich in vitamin C. However, in the process of making the juice, much is lost. In addition, most cranberry drinks on the market are a diluted product, reducing further the concentration of ascorbic acid (vitamin C). Although it would take a gallon or more of many cranberry drinks to contribute as much as one gram of ascorbic acid, the net result of drinking cranberry juice is still a slight degree of acidification. More important is the fact that the product can be used as a substitute for fruit drinks, fruit-ades and soda pops which tend to alkalinize the urine.

In addition to the above fluids, there are other foods that contribute to alkalinization of the urine. A list of these foods is included in the Appendix.

Many alcoholic beverages tend to alkalinize the urine. Although the immediate effect of alcohol consumption may be increased urinary output due to the fluid intake, inhibited antidiuretic hormone, and to dehydration of body tissues, the long-range effect is decreased urinary output as the body recovers from dehydration. During this period of reduced output the urine is concentrated, there is decreased bacterial washout and increased risk of crystalization of minerals.

To decrease calcium intake, dairy products are frequently limited for patients with long-term urinary problems. This restriction generally applies at least at the onset of their problem until it can be determined if the patient has a tendency to form stones.

APPLIANCES

Types of Catheters

A catheter is a tube which can be placed in the bladder to drain urine from the body. Indwelling catheters have a double lumen with an inflatable balloon at the tip (Fig. V-9).

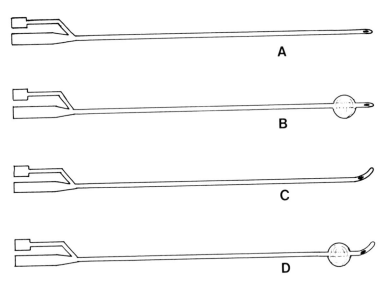

Figure V-9. Types of indwelling catheters. A. Foley catheter with balloon deflated. B. Foley catheter with balloon inflated. C. Coudé catheter with balloon deflated. D. Coudé catheter with balloon inflated.

For many years these catheters were made only of rubber or latex. Catheters now available are made either of solid silicone or of latex with a Teflon™ or silicone coating. Silicone or Teflon™ provides a smooth surface said to minimize irritation and catheter plugging.

Although both the solid and coated silicone catheters have the advantage of a smooth surface, there are some differences between the two types. The solid silicone catheter will not recover from a needle puncture, while the coated type, by virtue of the latex core, will seal itself. This is an important factor for patients requiring frequent urine cultures or bladder irrigation. If a sterile needle and syringe can be used to withdraw a specimen or instill a solution through the end of the catheter and it is not necessary to separate the catheter-tubing union, the chance of contamination of the drainage system or specimen is decreased (see "Catheter Irrigation" in this chapter).

This method cannot be used with the solid silicone catheters because they will leak from holes made by the needle punctures.

The walls of the solid silicone catheter are thinner and consequently have the advantage of a smaller diameter for the same size lumen as a comparable latex or coated latex catheter. With some patients this smaller size may cause less irritation. Since the solid silicone catheters are more expensive, these differences should be kept in mind when choosing a catheter for a patient.

Coudé catheters are made of a firmer material (e.g. red rubber) and have a curved tip. They are frequently used for difficult catheterization (Fig. V-9).

New products are constantly being produced, and it is well to keep informed about what is available and the advantages and disadvantages of these new products.

Catheter Sizes

Urethral indwelling catheters range in size from an French (Fr.) 8 to a Fr. 30. Sizes Fr. 14 or Fr. 16 are frequently used for adult patients, while smaller sizes are used for children. Catheters larger than Fr. 16 may be used for a patient who has problems with leakage around the catheter. It is best to use the smallest size that is functional to avoid unnecessary stretching of the urethra.

Catheters are available with either a 5-cc or a 30-cc inflatable balloon. Usually the 5-cc balloon is sufficient to keep the catheter in place. If a larger-sized balloon is required, a catheter with the 30-cc balloon may be used, with the balloon inflated only enough to keep the catheter in place, not necessarily to the full 30 cc.

Urine Collecting Appliances

Either an open or a closed urinary drainage system may be used with an indwelling catheter.

Open Drainage System

In the open drainage system, the catheter is packaged separately from the rest of the system and is attached to the urine collecting device after insertion. The catheter may be attached to a short tubing and leg bag for daytime use or to a longer tubing and collecting device for night or in bed use (Fig. V-10). The catheter and tubing are separated to change from one collecting device to another. It is this connecting, disconnecting and transferring procedure that has been cited as a frequent source of contamination.

An open drainage system is often used for long-term care or in a rehabili-

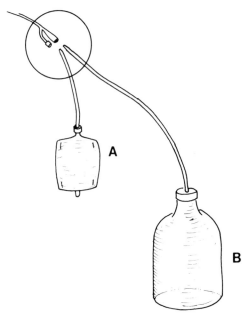

Figure V-10. Open drainage system. A. Day system with leg bag and short tubing. B. Night system with jug and longer tubing.

tation setting because of its convenience during patient activity. Clear plastic tubing is recommended, rather than opaque rubber or latex tubing, because the condition of the inside of the tubing is readily visible and because the smooth inside surface helps reduce the build up of extraneous material, mucus and bacterial growth. Most hospitals and many other health care facilities use new sterile equipment daily. However, for long-term or home care, the cost of new sterile equipment daily may become prohibitive. Disinfecting and reusing equipment for limited periods of time can be safe if proven procedures are followed meticulously.

Night Drainage System

Patients using leg bags during the day usually change to night drainage systems for bed. This system requires a longer tubing to facilitate placing the collecting device over the edge of the bed and a larger collecting apparatus to store urine over the longer period of time at night when output may be greater than in the daytime.

Care must be taken when selecting a receptacle for the urine collection, as it should be one that can be disinfected daily if reused. Many urine bags on the market have filters or drip chambers that make disinfection of the appliance difficult. We have found that the use of a night jug or bottle is a very effective, inexpensive option. The plastic bottles, in which distilled water is supplied, are ideal, as they are easily disinfected, lightweight and have a handle for attaching to the bed if desired.

The bottle or jug size needed will depend upon the anticipated nightly urinary output and the frequency with which it will be emptied during the night. The smaller the size used, the less solution will be required when it is disinfected, but it is important to be certain that it is big enough to prevent overflowing.

A two-holed rubber stopper fitted with an adapter in one hole will serve as a cap for the bottle and accommodate the tubing. The second hole serves as an air vent (Fig. V-11). Although this may seem like a rather primitive method for collecting urine overnight, it has proven to be both practical and economical for long-term use. The receptacle and its stopper can be easily washed and disinfected, thereby minimizing one source of infection.

The bottle or jug can be attached to the bed in the same manner as the conventional drainage bag or set on the floor inside a small box, wastebasket, or other receptacle that will prevent tipping (Fig. V-12).

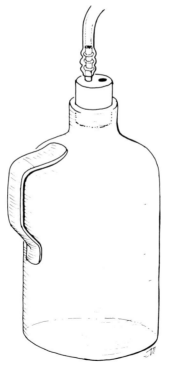

Figure V-11. Jug for night drainage collecting appliance with two-holed rubber stopper, adapter and tubing.

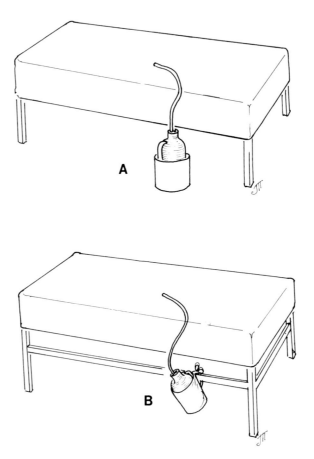

Figure V-12. Positioning of night drainage system using jug. A. Jug placed in receptacle to prevent tipping. B. Jug attached to bed.

Closed Drainage System

For a closed drainage system the catheter, tubing and urine collecting bag are packaged as one sterile unit (Fig. V-13). This unit is left intact during catheterization and at all times thereafter, eliminating the chance of contamination during the process of joining together separately packaged catheter, tubing and bag. If at any time the catheter-tubing union or tubing-bag union are separated, the system is no longer a closed system and the protocol for open-system care must be followed.

Closed drainage systems are usually used for short-term care and in the acute phase of an illness.

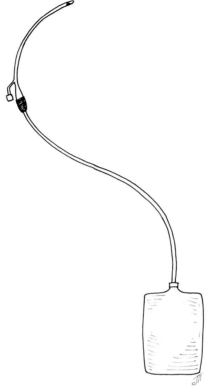

Figure V-13. Closed drainage system obtained sterile with catheter tubing and bag connected.

CARE PROCEDURES

Catheters may be obtained individually packaged or in kits containing some or all of the supplies necessary. Be sure to obtain all equipment needed before beginning to catheterize. Most health care facilities have established catheterization procedures making use of the types of supplies available in that facility. The procedure provided here is for a sterile "no-touch" technique.

Catheterization Procedures (No-Touch Method)

Supplies Needed

- Catheter kit (sterile catheter, sterile drape, sterile fenestrated drape, sterile forceps, lubricant, prefilled syringe to inflate balloon, sterile gloves, povidone-iodine swabs)
- extra pair of gloves (in case of contamination)
- extra sterile forceps
- Absorbent pads or washcloths
- Waterproof pads (e.g. Chux®)
- Detergent and water
- Non-sterile gloves
- Sterile syringe to deflate old catheter (sterile to avoid contamination should the balloon rupture)

Male Catheterization Procedure (No-Touch Method)

1. Reassure patient, explain what you are going to do, provide privacy.
2. Collect necessary materials. Place waste receptacle in an accessible place.
3. Wash hands.
4. Put on non-sterile gloves.
5. Place protective pad under patient's hips.
6. Using absorbent pads or washcloths, wash pubic area, perineum and genitalia, retracting foreskin to wash glans.
7. Remove non-sterile gloves.
8. Open kit using aseptic technique, using wrapper (sterile side up) as sterile cover for table.
9. Place drape near penis—(picking up by one corner, shake to open and place near penis).
10. Open second sterile forceps and place on sterile cover on table.
11. Put on sterile gloves.
12. Place fenestrated drape on sterile table cover.
13. Open povidone-iodine envelope and pour contents over sterile rayon balls.
14. Grasp penis with sterile drape, taking care not to contaminate hands.
15. Grasp rayon balls with forceps. Cleanse penis, starting with meatus and working down shaft. Pay special attention to cleansing base of glans and foreskin. Repeat three (3) times.
16. Release penis allowing it to lie on sterile drape while preparing catheter.

17. Using second "uncontaminated" sterile forceps, pick catheter out of tray and place it on sterile drape.
18. Open lubricant and lubricate catheter. Be sure to use sufficient lubricant to cover at least seven (7) inches of tip end of catheter.
19. Grasp penis with sterile drape and non-dominant hand, holding catheter with uncontaminated forceps, gently insert through meatus and slide through the urethra. DO NOT FORCE. If opposition is met, wait for sphincter to relax.
20. Insert catheter until urine flows (approximately 6–8 inches). Then, advance catheter another inch. Be sure catheter is draining well. If the catheter has a 5-cc balloon, inflate balloon with 7–10 cc sterile water. (If a 5-cc balloon catheter is not available and you are using a 30-cc balloon catheter, inflate balloon with 10 cc.)
21. Gently pull on catheter to obtain proper placement.
22. Wipe off excess povidone-iodine. (May use sterile drape to do this.)
23. Replace foreskin over glans in uncircumcised patient.
24. If a closed drainage system has been used, the drainage appliance (tubing and bag) will be already in place. Adjust it to be sure that there is a direct flow of urine away from the bladder into the collecting bag or, if an open system is used, attach tubing and leg bag or night bag to catheter using sterile procedure. (See Chapter XI, "Positioning Urinary Drainage Equipment.")
25. Remove all supplies.
26. Tape catheter firmly in place.
27. Check the appliance in 15 to 20 minutes to be sure urine is draining properly.

NOTE: If patient is allergic to povidone-iodine solution, repeat washing step.

Female Catheterization Procedure (No-Touch Method)

It is good to have a second person to assist in catheterization of a female patient to help hold legs in position. This is particularly important when catheterizing a paralyzed, immobilized or obese patient.

1. Reassure patient. Explain what you are going to do. Provide privacy.
2. Collect necessary materials. Place waste receptacle in accessible place.
3. Wash hands.
4. Put on non-sterile gloves.
5. Place protective pad under patient's hips.
6. Place patient in supine position. Spread patient's legs and raise knees. (Assistant can hold legs in place if necessary.)

7. Wash perineal area with soap and water.
8. Remove non-sterile gloves.
9. Open kit, using wrapper (sterile side up) as sterile cover for table.
10. Open second forceps and place on sterile field on table. Do not touch forceps.
11. Put on sterile gloves.
12. With sterile forceps, remove catheter from kit and place on sterile field.
13. Open lubricant and lubricate 3–4 inches at tip of catheter.
14. Open povidone-iodine solution and pour over rayon balls.
15. Open sterile drape and lay between patient's legs, close to perineum.
16. Open fenestrated paper and place over perineum with opening directly over labia.
17. With one gloved hand separate labia with thumb and index finger, working through hole in fenestrated paper. *DO NOT REMOVE THIS HAND. DO NOT* use this hand for sterile items thereafter. It is now contaminated.
18. Pick up rayon balls with sterile forceps and clean far side of labia in one downward stroke. Discard rayon ball. Wipe down near side with new rayon balls while keeping labia separated with thumb and index finger. *Wipe down center area with new rayon balls.* Repeat on both sides and center area.
19. Using sterile forceps with uncontaminated hand, pick up lubricated catheter and insert slowly and gently through urethral meatus until urine flows. Advance catheter about one inch further.
20. Inflate balloon with 7–10 cc sterile water. (Assistant can do this.)
21. Gently pull on catheter to attain proper placement.
22. If a "closed system" is being used, arrange tubing and collecting bag to allow urine to drain freely away from bladder. If an "open system" is used, attach sterile tubing leg bag or night collecting device to catheter using sterile procedure (see Chapter XI, "Positioning Urinary Drainage Equipment").
23. Dry perineum. Wipe off excess povidone-iodine.
24. Remove all equipment.
25. Tape catheter in place.
26. Check appliance in 15 to 20 minutes to be sure urine is draining properly.

NOTE: If patient is allergic to povidone-iodine solution, repeat washing step.

Taping the Catheter

It is important to tape the catheter firmly in place to prevent accidental pulling which could severely damage the bladder neck and urethra.

With a female, tape the catheter to the inner thigh (use adhesive tape unless patient is allergic) (Fig. V-14). With a male, tape the catheter with the penis in a somewhat upright position (Fig. V-14). This will minimize irritation in the penile-scrotal area, smooth out the urethral curve and eliminate pressure on the peno-scrotal junction which could lead to formation of a fistula. Enough slack should be left in the catheter to prevent tension and to accommodate an erection should it occur.

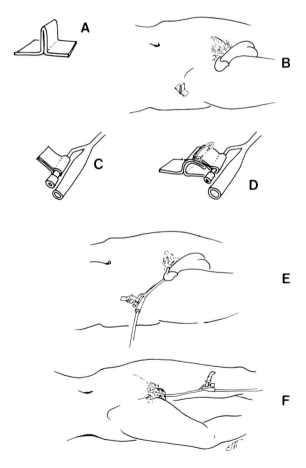

Figure V-14. Taping the catheter. A. Tape folded to make tab. B. Tab in place on abdomen. C. Tape attached to catheter. D. Catheter tape and tab pinned together. E. Catheter taped on male. F. Catheter taped on female.

Attach the tape to the catheter so that there are no kinks or sharp bends in the catheter to obstruct urine flow. Generally, it works well to place the tape on the balloon arm of the catheter rather than on the catheter itself. The catheter can then be attached, with a safety pin, to a small tab of tape placed on the abdomen in the male or inner thigh in the female (Fig. V-14). Occasionally, the physician may recommend a different position for taping.

Positioning of Drainage Appliances

The drainage tubing should always be placed so that there is a straight descending line from the bladder to the collecting appliance. See Chapter XI for detailed instructions and illustrations. The urine collecting appliance should always be below the level of the bladder.

Replacing Urinary Drainage Equipment

Catheters

When using an open drainage system the indwelling catheter should be changed at least once a month, even though it appears to be draining well. Bacteria growing inside the catheter are a source of contamination of the bladder. In addition, minerals tend to crystalize on the surface of the catheter, particularly on the balloon. As this shale sloughs off, it irritates the bladder mucosa and may form stones. The longer the catheter remains in place, the greater the risk of shale buildup. It is a good idea to cut open the tip of the old catheter and examine it for granular material. If present, it should be reported to the physician.

Tubing, Leg Bags and Night Drainage System

When using an open drainage system a fresh sterile or disinfected tubing, leg bag and night collecting system should be used daily (see Chapter XI, "Disinfecting Procedure").

Ideally, reused disinfected tubing and bags should be replaced with new, sterile equipment once a week. If this is not financially possible, the equipment should be replaced at two-week intervals or at least once a month.

Closed Drainage System

With a closed drainage system, it is recommended that the entire system (i.e. catheter, tubing and bag) be changed at least every one to two weeks.

Since a catheterized patient will always eventually develop bacteriuria, the tubing and bag, if used longer, will become heavily colonized with bacteria and be a constant source of reinfection.

All Drainage Appliances

If a patient is being treated for a urinary tract infection, all new catheter, tubing and drainage bags should be used after treatment has progressed five to seven days and before treatment is completed to eliminate the chance of reinfection from contaminated equipment.

Catheter Irrigation

For many years it was routine policy to irrigate an indwelling catheter once or twice a day, whether the catheter was plugging or not. In recent years, it has been found that this irrigation is usually not necessary and may wash bacteria into the bladder. A fluid intake sufficient to provide an output of 2,000 to 3,000 ml/day is sufficient to provide "self-irrigation" of the catheter.

If it is necessary to irrigate because the catheter is plugging with mucus or granular material, extreme care must be taken to minimize the chance of bacterial contamination as well as to avoid tissue damage from too vigorous irrigation.

An open or closed method of irrigation may be used and the choice will depend upon the equipment available and the type of indwelling catheter in use.

In the open method of irrigation, the catheter is separated from the collecting tubing and the irrigating solution is allowed to flow into the bladder through the open end of the catheter by gravity. Never use force. The closed method provides for irrigating without separating the catheter-tubing union. The irrigation solution is instilled into the bladder through the catheter at the catheter-tubing union using a 24-gauge needle and syringe. The small-gauge needle will prevent too forceful a stream against the bladder wall. This method cannot be used with solid silicone catheters, as they will leak through the needle punctures.

Irrigation through a special three-way catheter is used only under special circumstances and will not be discussed.

Health care facilities frequently have their own protocols and procedures using equipment available at the facilities. Procedures for open and closed drainage systems and a list of supplies needed for these procedures are also included here.

Catheter Irrigation (Open Method)

Supplies Needed
- Catheter irrigation kit (sterile irrigation syringe, sterile jar or glass, sterile measure, sterile basin, forceps or clamp, alcohol wipes)

NOTE: If a kit is used, check carefully to be sure all necessary supplies are included. Contents of kits vary.

- Sterile gauze pads
- Rubber band
- Non-sterile gloves
- Sterile irrigation solution as prescribed. (This is usually a buffered acidic solution, e.g. Renacidin® or Solution G®.)
- Sterile normal saline
- Waterproof pad (e.g. Chux®)

Procedure (Fig. V-15)
1. Explain to patient what you are going to do; provide privacy.
2. Obtain all necessary supplies.
3. Wash hands vigorously.
4. Put on non-sterile gloves.
5. Place waterproof pad or towel under patient's hips.
6. Wipe neck of bottle of solution with alcohol wipes to remove any dust particles.
7. Pour the prescribed amount (usually 30 ml) of irrigating solution into sterile measuring glass and saline into sterile jar (Fig. V-15A).
8. Wipe catheter-tubing union well with alcohol wipes and place the sterile basin under the catheter (Fig. V-15B).
9. Clamp the catheter above the catheter-tubing union and disconnect the tubing from the catheter (Fig. V-15B).
10. Cover open end of tubing with sterile gauze and secure with a rubber band (Fig. V-15C).
11. Insert tip of syringe (without bulb or plunger) into catheter, being careful not to touch the end of the catheter or tip of syringe (Fig. V-15D).
12. Pour irrigating solution into open end of syringe (Fig. V-15E).
13. Release clamp and allow solution to flow into bladder by gravity.
14. Clamp catheter and remove syringe; allow solution to remain in the bladder the prescribed length of time (usually, 20 to 30 minutes).
15. Unclamp and allow bladder to empty and the solution to flow out into sterile basin (Fig. V-13F).

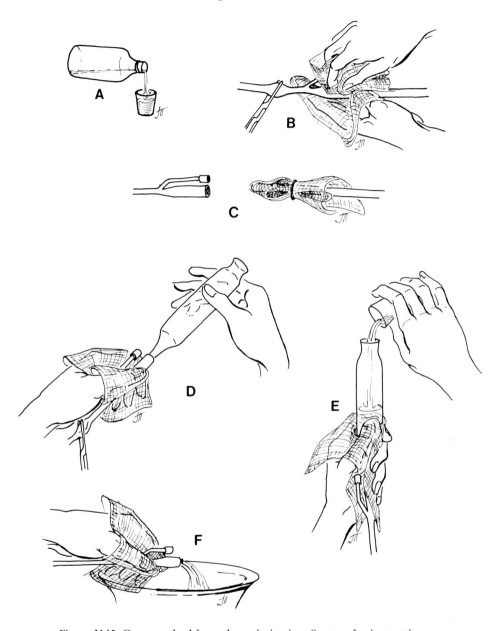

Figure V-15. Open method for catheter irrigation. See text for instructions.

16. If an additional irrigation with sterile saline is to be used, reinsert syringe into catheter and clamp catheter.
17. Pour the prescribed amount (usually 30 ml) of sterile saline into syringe. Release clamp and allow saline to flow into bladder by gravity.

18. Allow bladder to empty and saline to flow out into sterile pan.
19. Wipe ends of catheter and tubing with alcohol wipes and reconnect.
20. Adjust appliance so all equipment is properly placed.
21. Remove non-sterile gloves and wash hands.

If a patient's bladder is to be irrigated on a regular basis, the same bottle of irrigating solution may be used for up to one week provided it is refrigerated between use. Do not reuse the same bottle of irrigating solution for more than one patient. Do not reuse open bottles of sterile saline, as saline will support bacterial growth. To avoid waste, it is best to obtain these solutions in small-sized bottles.

Catheter Irrigation (Closed Method)

NOTE: This method cannot be used with solid silicone catheters because they will leak at the site of needle puncture. The puncture sites of latex and Teflon or silicone-coated latex catheters will seal themselves.

Supplies Needed

- Sterile syringe—50 cc
- Sterile 24-gauge needle
- Sterile medicine glass or jar
- Alcohol wipes or 70 percent alcohol and sterile gauze pads
- Kelly clamp—forceps
- Irrigation solution as prescribed by physician
- Sterile irrigation saline if prescribed by physician

Procedure (Fig. V-16)

1. Obtain all necessary materials.
2. Wash hands.
3. Put on non-sterile gloves.
4. Vigorously wipe the irrigation site with alcohol wipes and leave alcohol wipe covering irrigation site. (Fig. V-16A)
5. Prepare syringe for irrigation. Attach sterile 24 gauge needle to the sterile syringe.
6. Wipe cap and shoulder of irrigation solution bottles with alcohol to remove any dust particles.
7. Pour solution into sterile glass or jar. (fig. V-16B)
8. Withdraw 30 cc, or amount prescribed, of solution into syringe. Be careful not to contaminate the solution or needle. (Fig. V-16C)

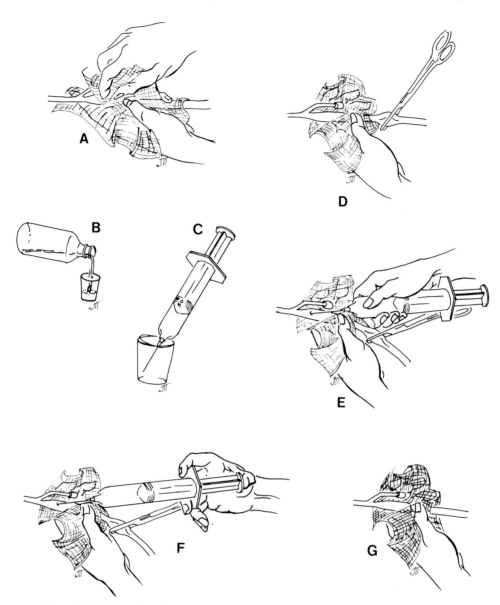

Figure V-16. Closed method for catheter irrigation. See text for instructions.

9. Clamp tubing just below irrigation site and rub catheter-tubing union with alcohol wipe again. (fig. V-16D)
10. Insert needle into catheter-irrigation site. Be careful not to insert the needle through both sides of the catheter. *Always insert the needle below the inflating tubing* (Fig. V-16E).
11. Slowly instill the irrigating solution by pushing in the plunger of the

syringe. Fluid will not flow in by gravity through the 24-gauge needle. The pressure used to force the fluid through the needle will not be so great as to damage the bladder (Fig. V-16F).

12. Withdraw the needle and wipe site with the alcohol wipe (Fig. V-16G).
13. Release the clamp and allow the solution to drain out of the bladder or leave the clamp in place for the prescribed period of time. Then release clamp and allow bladder to empty.
14. If ordered, the bladder can be flushed with sterile saline solution after the irrigation solution flush. Follow the same procedure as for the irrigation solution. Be sure to wipe the neck of the saline bottle with alcohol wipes before pouring.
15. After completion of irrigation, arrange collection appliance and retape catheter if it was necessary to untape before the procedure.
16. Remove all equipment.
17. Take off non-sterile gloves and wash hands.

If a patient is to be irrigated on a regular basis, the same bottle of irrigating solution may be used for up to one week provided it is refrigerated between use. Do not reuse the same bottle of irrigating solution for more than one patient. Do not reuse open bottles of sterile saline, as saline will support bacterial growth. To avoid waste, it is best to obtain these solutions in small-sized bottles.

IMPORTANT THINGS TO REMEMBER ABOUT INDWELLING URETHRAL CATHETER DRAINAGE

1. Always wash hands before and after drainage appliance care.
2. Use sterile procedure to catheterize the patient.
3. Be sure to cleanse catheter-tubing union with alcohol or povidone-iodine before separating. Do not use fingertips or fingernails directly on catheter or tubing.
4. Cover any open ends of tubing or catheter with sterile gauze pads. Do not touch open ends.
5. Do not allow urine to flow back toward bladder from tubing and urine collection device.
6. Always place drainage tubing in descending line from bladder to urine collecting appliance.
7. Cleanse perineal area and exposed catheter twice daily.
8. Tape catheter securely in place.
9. Use new sterile or disinfected drainage equipment daily (e.g. tubing, leg bag, night bag or jug).

10. Encourage good fluid intake and urine acidification.

E.N.

REFERENCES

1. Wershub, L.P: *Urology: From Antiquity to the Twentieth Century.* St. Louis, Warren H. Green, Inc., 1970.
2. Stamm, W.E.: Guidelines for prevention of catheter associated urinary tract infections. *Ann Int Med 82:*386–390, 1975.
3. Kass, E.H., and Schneideman, L.J.: Entry of bacteria into the urinary tracts of patients with indwelling catheters. *N Eng J Med 256:*556–557, 1957.
4. Burke, J.P., Jacobson, J.A., Garibaldi, R.A., Conti, M.T., and Alling, D.W.: Evaluation of daily meatal care with poly-antibiotic ointment in prevention of urinary catheter-associated bacteriuria. *J Urol 129:*331–334, 1983.
5. Price, M., and Newman, E.: Factors associated with deterioration of kidney function in patients with spinal cord injury. *JAMWA 29:*67–70, 1974.
6. Lome, L.G., and Navani, S.: Foley calculus formation. *Br J Radiol 43:*487–488, 1970.
7. Kaufman, J.M., Fam, B., Jacobs, S.C., Gabilondo, F., Yalla, S., Kane, J.P., and Rossier, A.B.: Bladder cancer and squamous metaplasia in spinal cord injury patients. *J Urol 118:*967–971, 1977.
8. Newman, D.M., Brown, J.R., Jay, A.C., and Pontius, E.E.: Squamous cell carcinoma of the bladder. *J Urol 100:*470–473, 1968.
9. Boyarsky, S.: Bladder cancer and spinal cord injured patients. (Letter to the editor.) *Urol 15:*639, 1980.
10. Devenport, J.K., Swenson, J.R., Dukes, G.E., and Sonsalla, P.K.: Formaldehyde generation from methenamine salts in spinal cord injury. *Arch Phys Med Rehabil 65:*257–259, 1984.

Chapter VI

SUPRAPUBIC CATHETERS

One of the earliest reports of the use of a suprapubic catheter for the management of a neurogenic bladder is the 1917 report by Thomson Walker, a surgeon to King George Hospital in England.[1] He reported the use of suprapubic cystotomy to drain the bladder of spinal cord injured soldiers. It was his belief that this method of drainage would prevent tension within the bladder, decrease ascending infection and preserve the urethra. At that time, indwelling urethral catheters had to be tied or taped to retain them within the bladder.

Suprapubic cystotomy was for many years the treatment of choice in the management of spinal cord injury.[2] With the development of the self-retaining catheter, indwelling urethral catheter drainage became more popular.

Suprapubic bladder drainage is also used frequently during certain surgical procedures and in obstetrics. This is usually accomplished using a smaller-sized catheter tubing (Nos. 8 or 10) and is used for short duration.[3] Long-term suprapubic drainage using the larger-size self-retaining catheters (e.g. Fr. 24 or Fr. 26) is accomplished through a surgical procedure (Fig. VI-1).

NOTE: Many of the problems, dangers and procedures for suprapubic catheter drainage are similar to those of indwelling urethral catheter drainage. In the interest of space, the reader is referred to Chapter V "Indwelling Catheters" frequently throughout this chapter.

INDICATIONS FOR USE

Indications for use of a suprapubic catheter are similar to those for use of an indwelling urethral catheter, namely, incontinence or the inability to void (see Chap. V, "Indications for Use").

If an indwelling catheter is required, the decision of whether to use an indwelling urethral or suprapubic catheter will be made by the clinician and patient. A suprapubic catheter may be the method of choice if there has been urethral scarring, urethral diverticulum or strictures, or other damage to the urethra making indwelling urethral catheterization inadvisable.

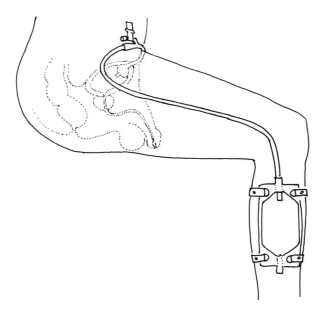

Figure VI-1. Suprapubic catheter placed through the abdominal wall into the bladder by a surgical procedure.

Suprapubic catheter drainage is sometimes provided for the sexually active patient to eliminate the presence of a urethral catheter during intercourse, although not all physicians agree that this is a legitimate reason for performing suprapubic insertion. Sexual intercourse is possible with an indwelling urethral catheter in place, but, in either sex, it can cause urethral trauma.

Our research has shown that with carefully managed long-term care, there has been no difference in rate of change of kidney function in patients using indwelling urethral catheters and suprapubic catheters.[4]

INHERENT DANGERS

Infection, calculi and mechanical tissue damage are three major factors contributing to the inherent dangers of suprapubic drainage.

Infection

As with indwelling urethral catheters, bacteriuria is a common occurrence with long-term suprapubic drainage. It is important then to keep the bacteria within the bladder from invading the bladder wall, resulting in cystitis and from reaching the kidneys where they can cause pyelonephritis.

This can best be accomplished by discouraging bacterial growth with an acid urine, maintaining an adequate washout with a good fluid intake, and by preventing damage to tissue within the urinary tract.

Fluid intake, diet and urine acidification will be discussed later in the chapter. The organism isolation pattern will be discussed in Chapter XI.

Danger Areas

Three main danger areas exist where bacteria can enter the system: the stoma site, the catheter-tubing union and the collecting applicance (see Fig. VI-2).

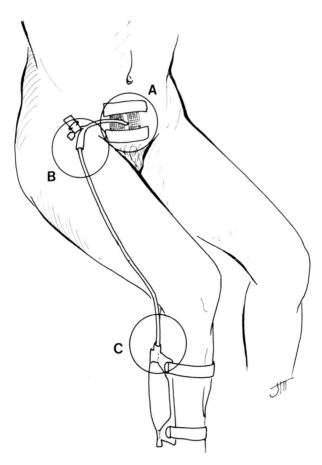

Figure VI-2. Danger areas where bacteria can enter the system. A. Stoma site. B. Catheter-tubing union. C. Tubing and urine collecting appliance.

Stoma Site: Care must be taken during initial catheterization. All hair must be removed from directly around the stoma to prevent it from being pushed into the bladder by the catheter. The site should be carefully cleansed before catheterizing and twice daily thereafter with povidone-iodine or a detergent and water. If there is a large amount of purulent material or bleeding at the stoma site, this should be reported to the physician. It is important to cleanse the exposed catheter itself to remove mucus and crusty material. Covering the stoma site with fresh sterile gauze pads twice daily will help keep the area clean and reduce the risk of infection (Fig. VI-2A)

Catheter-Tubing Union: The catheter-tubing union is a frequent source of bacterial contamination (Fig. VI-2B). The fingernails and fingertips should not come into direct contact with the catheter and tubing during separation. Vigorously wipe the catheter-tubing union site with alcohol wipes and then hold catheter and tubing with wipes while separating. The open ends of the catheter and tubing should always be covered with alcohol wipes or sterile gauze pads until reconnected. See Chapter V for illustrations of correct procedure.

Tubing and Urine Collecting Device: The third danger area is the tubing and urine collecting device (Fig. VI-2C). The importance of daily disinfection and frequent replacement of equipment has already been discussed. The leg bag or night bag must always be kept below the level of the bladder, with the tubing in a straight, descending position (Figs. VI-3 & VI-4). When transferring the collecting appliance from one area to another, the tubing should be clamped or pinched to prevent urine from flowing back into the bladder. See Chapter XI for complete instructions on care and positioning of appliances.

Calculi

Patients with long-term catheterization, whether suprapubic or urethral, are at risk to develop bladder or renal calculi. Conditions favorable to the development of calculi have been discussed in Chapters IV and V. Special emphasis should be placed on several factors for patients with suprapubic catheters.

1. *The high incidence of bacteriuria:* Bacteria form a nidus upon which minerals from a supersaturated solution can crystalize.

2. *The presence of a foreign body within the bladder:* The catheter itself forms a nidus upon which minerals can crystalize.

3. *Stagnant urine within the bladder:* The suprapubic catheter is inserted through the top of the bladder allowing urine to pool in the bladder neck where urine may become supersaturated, allowing minerals to crystalize.

Sufficient, consistent fluid intake, frequent catheter changes, numerous

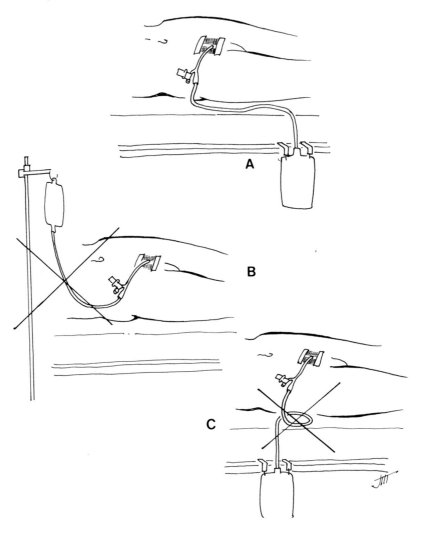

Figure VI-3. Urine collecting system for suprapubic catheter. A. Correctly placed. B. Incorrectly placed above level of bladder. C. Incorrectly placed with loop in tubing.

position changes by the patient and urine acidification will help minimize calculus formation.

Mechanical Damage

Mechanical damage to the suprapubic stoma can occur during passage of the catheter if adequate lubrication is not provided or if the catheter is too large for the stoma opening. The catheter should be inserted well inside the bladder before the balloon is inflated.

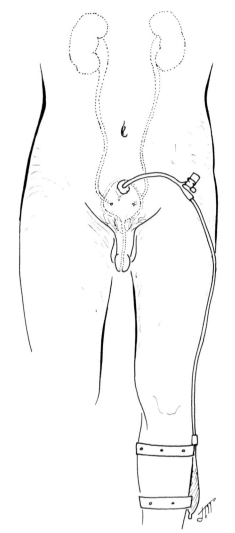

Figure VI-4. Suprapubic catheter with tubing and leg bag correctly placed.

Tissue damage may occur at the stoma site if the catheter is inadvertently pulled, forcing the balloon against the bladder wall or even into the stoma. Anchoring the catheter to the abdomen will minimize the danger (see "Care Procedure").

Overdistention of the bladder may result from a plugged or kinked catheter or tubing or from a full collecting appliance. Acute overdistention can result in septicemia if bacteria gain entrance into the bloodstream through ruptured capillaries and larger blood vessels. Chronic or recurrent overdistention leads to the development of bladder diverticula and vesicoureteral reflux.

Crystals, shale and calculi frequently irritate the bladder wall causing hematuria and providing a site for bacterial invasion with resultant cystitis or systemic infection.

EFFECT OF DIET AND FLUID INTAKE

Unless medically contraindicated, fluid intake should be sufficient to insure an output of at least 2500 ml per day. Remember that most bacteria causing urinary tract infections multiply by cell division at the rate of one division each 20 to 30 minutes. It is, therefore, important that there be adequate fluid intake at periodic intervals to insure a continual washing out of the bacteria present. Water and cranberry juice are generally the best fluids to drink. The merits of cranberry juice are discussed in Chapter V, "The Effect of Diet and Fluid Intake." When attempting to increase fluid intake, it is important to keep in mind the fact that citrus fruit juices, fruit drinks (ades) and soda pops tend to alkalinize the urine. Other foods which have an alkaline ash are listed in the Appendix.

Alcoholic beverages should be discouraged for patients with long-term urinary problems. Many alcoholic beverages tend to alkalinize the urine and cause dehydration of body tissues. This dehydration will result in an initial increase in urinary output followed by a long-range decrease in urinary output as the body recovers from dehydration. During the period of reduced output, the urine may become quite concentrated with a decrease in bacterial washout and an increased risk of crystalization of minerals present in the urine.

Although the effect of diet upon calcium excretion is controversial, dairy products are frequently limited for patients with long-term urinary drainage problems. Restrictions are usually continued until it can be determined if the patient has a tendency to form stones.

Medications are sometimes given to acidify the urine (see Chapter V, "Effect of Diet and Fluid Intake").

APPLIANCES

Types of Catheters

Except for their size, the catheters generally now used for suprapubic drainage are the same types as those used for indwelling urethral drainage. They may be either latex, latex with silicone or Teflon coating, or solid silicone. Both the solid silicone and the Teflon or silicone coated have the advantage of having a smooth surface which tends to minimize problems with catheters plugging. Since the walls of the solid silicone catheter are thinner, the outside diameter is smaller in relation to the size of lumen than for latex or coated latex catheters. This is not particularly important with suprapubic placement, as the stoma will close around the catheter and prevent leakage. It should be remembered that the needle-syringe method cannot be used to irrigate or withdraw urine from solid silicone catheters, as they will not recover from needle puncture.

At one time, the Malecot® catheter was frequently used for suprapubic drainage. It was a catheter that had winged projections on the end to retain it within the bladder (Fig. VI-5). A stylet placed inside the catheter was used to stretch the tip of the catheter to flatten the wings during insertion. The catheter was removed by forceful pulling to compress the wings, often producing bleeding from the stoma site. The Malecot catheter has largely been replaced by the less traumatic balloon retention catheter.

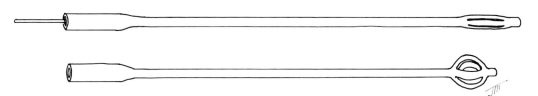

Figure VI-5. Malecot catheter. A. With stylet in place for insertion. B. With stylet removed and wings expanded.

Catheter Size

Larger-size catheters are generally used for suprapubic drainage to prevent closure of the stoma and to minimize problems with the catheter plugging. In adult patients, the sizes most frequently used are a Fr. 24 or Fr. 26, often with a 30-cc balloon rather than a 5-cc balloon, to insure that the catheter will remain in the bladder. It is usually not necessary to inflate the balloon to the full 30 cc, with 10 or 15 cc being sufficient.

If the stoma opening is small, it may be necessary to use a smaller catheter; however, the size of the opening can be enlarged by gradually increasing the size of the catheter. For example, if delay is encountered in replacing a suprapubic catheter, the stoma may close and it will be necessary to use a catheter several sizes smaller. Thereafter, at monthly intervals, each time the catheter is changed, one size larger can be used until the original size is attained. The physician should be informed of the necessity for using a smaller catheter and asked for approval to gradually increase the size. Do not delay the placement of the smaller catheter until the physician can be contacted, as the stoma may close completely.

Urine Collecting Devices

Open drainage systems are usually used with suprapubic catheterizations because closed drainage kits with larger than Fr. 18 catheters are not now commercially available. If the catheter is packaged separately from the tubing and urine collection appliance and the parts must be connected before use, the system is called an *open drainage system.* Only those systems that are obtained sterile with all units connected are referred to as a *closed drainage system.* If the parts are disconnected at any time for any reason, the system is no longer a closed system.

Open Drainage System

With an open drainage system the catheter may be attached to a short tubing and leg bag for daytime use or to a longer tubing and night drainage bag or jug. This method of drainage necessitates separating the catheter from the tubing to transfer from night to day drainage. It is in the process of separating the catheter and tubing that contamination of the system may occur.[5] It was because of this long recognized source of contamination that the closed drainage system was developed.

Even if a closed system were available with the size catheter required, an open system is often preferred to allow the patient to use a leg bag for daytime use and for convenience during patient activities and recreational functions.

Clear plastic tubing is recommended rather than rubber tubing because the condition of the inside of the tubing is readily visible and because the smooth inside surface helps reduce buildup of extraneous material, mucus and bacterial growth (see Chap. V, "Open Drainage System").

Night Drainage System

The night drainage system will be the same as with indwelling urethral catheters (see Chap. V, "Night Drainage System").

Closed drainage systems generally are not used with suprapubic drainage. If in use, the system will be the same as for indwelling catheters (see Chap. V, "Closed Drainage System").

CARE PROCEDURES

Be sure to obtain all the necessary supplies before removing the old catheter. The suprapubic stoma may close quite rapidly after the catheter is removed.

Most health care facilities have established procedures making use of the types of supplies available in that facility. The procedures provided here are for a sterile no-touch method of catheterization.

Suprapubic Catheterization Procedure (Sterile "No Touch")

Supplies Needed

- Catheter kit, plus correct size catheter and pre-filled syringe (sterile catheter, pre-filled syringe, sterile drape, sterile fenestrated drape, sterile forceps, lubricant, sterile gloves, povidone-iodine swabs or solution and sterile rayon balls)
- extra pair of sterile gloves (in case of contamination)
- extra sterile forceps
- Waterproof pad (e.g. Chux®)
- Detergent and water
- Non-sterile gloves
- Razor—to shave around stoma site if necessary
- Sterile 10-cc syringe to deflate balloon of old catheter (sterile to avoid contamination should the balloon rupture)

Procedure

1. Reassure patient, explain what you are going to do, and provide privacy.
2. Collect all necessary materials, place waste receptacle in an accessible place.
3. Wash hands.
4. Put on non-sterile gloves (for your own protection as well as patient's).
5. Place protective pad over patient's abdomen below level of stoma.
6. Using absorbent pads or washcloth, wash around stoma site. Remove all caked, crusty material.
7. Shave any hair growing close to stoma site. Wipe away all loose hairs to avoid pushing them into bladder with catheter.
8. If crusty or mucous material still remains around stoma, wash again with detergent and water.

9. Open catheter kit using aseptic technique. Use wrapper as table cover, placing sterile side up.
10. Open package and place second sterile forcep on sterile drape on table. Do not touch forcep.
11. Open catheter and place on sterile cover on table. Do not touch catheter.
12. Deflate balloon of catheter and remove catheter, laying it across pad on abdomen.
13. Remove non-sterile gloves and put on sterile gloves.
14. Open povidone-iodine envelope and pour contents over sterile rayon balls.
15. Grasp rayon balls with forceps. Cleanse stoma site starting at center and working outwards in circular manner. Repeat three times.
16. Place fenestrated drape on abdomen with opening over stoma site.
17. Open lubricant and lubricate catheter. Be sure to use enough lubricant to cover at least four inches of tip end of catheter.
18. Using second sterile forcep, pick up catheter and gently pass tip of catheter through stoma site into bladder. You may encounter some resistance, particularly if patient's bladder is spastic. Wait a few seconds for muscles to relax and try again with gentle pressure. (If continued resistance is encountered, it may be necessary to use a smaller-size catheter.) Insert catheter until urine flows freely, then continue to insert about one inch further.
19. Using pre-filled syringe, inflate balloon with 7 to 10 cc of sterile water.
20. *Gently* pull on catheter to obtain proper placement.
21. Attach sterile tubing and urine collecting appliance, being careful to avoid contamination.
22. Gently wash around stoma site to remove excess lubricant and povidone-iodine solution.
23. Place sterile gauze pad around stoma site. Fold pad in half, place one on either side of catheter and tape (see Fig. VI-2).
24. Tape catheter to abdomen (see Fig. VI-2).
25. Remove sterile gloves.
26. Remove all equipment and dispose of properly.
27. Wash hands.

NOTE: If patient is allergic to povidone-iodine solution, repeat washing step.

You may notice that there is a pink tinge to urine and a few small clots in the first urine passed; this is not unusual. However, excessive bleeding should be reported to the physician and patient observed until bleeding ceases or there has been medical intervention.

Always check appliance about 20–30 minutes after insertion to be sure urine is draining properly.

Remember, when changing a suprapubic catheter, you will want to work quickly because the stoma openings tend to close quite rapidly. Have everything ready before removing the old catheter. If it has been necessary to use a smaller size catheter, the physician should be informed.

Taping of Catheter

The suprapubic catheter should be taped firmly in place to prevent accidental pulling. Tape the catheter to the abdomen with enough slack to prevent pulling with position changes. It should be placed so that clothing (e.g. belt) will not obstruct urine flow and so there are no sharp kinks or bends. The exact placement will vary with body configuration (Fig. VI-4).

Positioning Drainage Appliance

The drainage tubing should always be placed so there is a straight descending line from the stoma site to the collecting appliance. See Chapter XI, "Positioning of Urinary Drainage Equipment," for detailed instructions and illustrations.

Replacing Urinary Drainage Equipment

Catheters

Suprapubic catheters should be changed once a month even though they appear to be draining well. Catheters left in for longer periods of time often will adhere to the tissue within the stoma and produce trauma when removed. The catheters tend to become coated inside and out with mucus or other extraneous material, providing an environment for bacterial growth and mineral crystalization. It is a good idea to cut open the tip of the used catheter and examine it for granular material. If present, this should be reported to the physician.

Tubing, Leg Bags and Night Drainage Systems

When using the "open system of drainage," a fresh sterile or disinfected tubing, leg bag and night drainage system should be used every day (see Chapter XI, "Disinfection Procedure").

Ideally, the tubing and bags should be replaced with new sterile equipment once a week. If this is not financially possible, do so at two-week intervals or at least once a month.

If a patient is being treated for a urinary tract infection, all new equipment (i.e. catheter, tubing, bags) should be used after treatment has progressed five to seven days and before treatment is completed to eliminate the chance of reinfection from contaminated equipment.

Catheter Irrigation

Irrigation of the suprapubic catheter is usually not necessary, and this extra manipulation of the catheter may, in fact, contribute to contamination of the system. A fluid intake sufficient to provide an output of 2500 to 3000 ml/day is usually sufficient to provide "self-irrigation" of the catheter.

If irrigation is necessary because of catheter plugging, extreme care must be taken to avoid contamination and tissue damage. See Chapter V for irrigation procedure.

Stoma Site

The stoma site should be cleaned twice daily with povidone-iodine or detergent and water to remove any secretions. Be sure to clean the exposed catheter to remove any crusty material which may harbor bacteria and irritate the tissue. Occasionally, the tissue around the stoma may become infected. Check carefully for any indications of infection. If present, this should be reported to the physician.

IMPORTANT THINGS TO REMEMBER ABOUT SUPRAPUBIC CATHETERS

1. Always wash hands vigorously before and after urinary drainage appliance care.
2. Use sterile procedure to insert the catheter.
3. Be sure to cleanse catheter-tubing union area with alcohol or povidone-iodine before separating. Do not use fingertips or fingernails directly on the catheter and tubing.
4. Cover any open ends of tubing and catheter with a sterile gauze pad. Do not touch open ends.
5. Do not allow urine to flow back towards bladder from tubing and urine collecting device.
6. Always place drainage tubing in descending line from bladder to urine collecting device.

7. Cleanse around stoma area and exposed catheter twice daily. Check for any indication of infection in tissue around stoma.
8. Tape catheter securely in place.
9. Use new sterile or disinfected drainage equipment daily (i.e. tubing, leg bag, night bag or jug).
10. Encourage good fluid intake and urine acidification.

E.N.

REFERENCES

1. Thomson Walker, J.W.: The bladder of gunshot and other injuries of the spinal cord. *Lancet 1:*173–177, 1917.
2. Cook, J.B., and Smith, P.H.: Percutaneous suprapubic cystostomy after spinal cord injury. *Br J Urol 48:*119–121, 1976.
3. Peloso, O.A., Wilkinson, L.H., and Floyd, V.T.: Suprapubic bladder drainage in general surgery. *Arch Surg 106:*568–572, 1973.
4. Price, M.: Some results of a fifteen year vertical study of urinary function in spinal cord injured patients: A preliminary report. *J Am Para Soc 5:*31–34, 1982.
5. Desautels, R.E.: The causes of catheter induced urinary infection and their prevention. *J Urol 101:*757–760, 1969.

Chapter VII

EXTERNAL CATHETERS

An external catheter is a device which attaches over the penis to collect urine and drain it into a collecting appliance. Sometimes referred to as condom or sheath drainage, these appliances are available in a variety of styles and sizes. Satisfactory external catheters are currently available for male patients only. It is hoped that reliable external catheters will soon be developed for female patients.

Early appliances were quite primitive compared to those currently in use. Some consisted of rubber bags into which the penis was placed. The bag was then attached to the body by means of straps or tape. This was later improved to more snugly fitting bags and finally to the use of a condom.[1,2] Although external catheters made from a condom are still used by some patients, there are several other types commercially available. We will briefly discuss the use of each of these types. The need of each patient varies and the type that works well for one person may be unsatisfactory for another. It is good to be aware of the advantages and disadvantages of each type when choosing an appliance.

INDICATIONS FOR USE

The primary reason for using an external catheter is incontinence whether this is due to spontaneous uncontrollable voiding or due to intermittent or continuous leaking. External catheters are also used by male patients who are able to void, either voluntarily or by triggering a reflex bladder contraction, but who for some reason, such as urgency or decreased manual dexterity, are unable to use a urinal or toilet.

The number of patients using external catheters has increased markedly with the development of better care procedures and improvement in results of surgical procedures.

Surgical Procedures

Sphincterotomy

Failure of the external sphincter to relax when there is a detrusor bladder contraction is referred to as *dyssynergia*. This results in increased pressure within the bladder with failure to expel the urine. The increased pressure can result in bladder diverticula, reflux and hydronephrosis. A surgical procedure can be performed in which the sphincter muscle is cut (*sphincterotomy*), allowing the urine to flow with or without bladder contraction. This procedure formerly resulted in impotency in some patients. Newer techniques have reduced this complication to less than 10 percent. When performing sphincterotomies, conservative incisions are made to minimize bleeding. Occasionally, the sphincterotomy will have to be repeated, either because the first approach was too conservative or because scar tissue has reduced the effectiveness of the procedure. Since this is a permanent form of intervention and the patient will always be incontinent, it is usually not performed until other methods of management (e.g. pharmacological) have been tried.[3]

Penile Prosthesis

Penile prostheses were first devised as an aid in the management of impotence.[4] In patients with a neurogenic bladder, penile prosthesis may also be used to enable the more satisfactory use of an external catheter. There are several different types of prostheses, rigid or semi-rigid rods or inflatable rods implanted into the corpora cavernosa. The prosthesis adds length, girth and stability to the penis, permitting an easier, more dependable attachment of an external catheter.[5] These patients require continued close follow-up because of dangers of protrusion and compression of the urethra or of bladder neck outlet obstruction. Sometimes, a sphincterotomy is needed to allow free outflow of urine.

Both the patient and sex partner should be informed of physiological and psychological implications of the procedure.

INHERENT DANGERS

There are five major problems or dangers that can result from the use of an external catheter: *infection, calculi, bladder overdistention, vesicoureteral reflux,* and *mechanical damage.*

Infection

Males using the non-invasive external catheter could be expected to have fewer urinary tract infections than those utilizing an indwelling urethral or suprapubic catheter. However, statistics have belied this hypothesis. We have found that 63 percent of our population of spinal cord injured patients using external catheters returned for annual follow-up with bacteriuria.[6]

There are several factors that may contribute to bacteriuria in these patients. Urine pooling within the external catheter will allow bacteria present to multiply and migrate through the urethra into the bladder. The rate of growth (multiplication) of the bacteria will be influenced by the pH of the urine. (Most bacteria causing urinary tract infections grow best in a neutral or alkaline pH.) The incidence of infection will also be affected by the volume of residual urine, that is, the amount of urine remaining in the bladder after a triggered or spontaneous void.[7,8]

Danger Areas

There are three major danger areas where bacteria may enter the system with external catheter drainage: the perineal area, the tubing, and the urine collecting appliance (Fig. VII-1).

Perineal Area and Sheath: Cleanliness of self and appliance are essential to minimize bacterial contamination (Fig. VII-1A). Obstructed flow of urine from the bladder caused by kinking and twisting of the sheath can lead to overdistention of the bladder and back pressure to the kidneys (Fig. VII-2). Pooling of urine in the sheath will permit bacterial migration through the urethra to the bladder. Improper application of appliance can result in tissue breakdown because of pressure or abrasion.

Tubing: Obstruction or kinking of the tubing will lead to accumulation of urine within the sheath and eventually to back pressure and overdistention (Fig. VII-1B). Improper handling of the tubing and collection bag will permit a backflow of urine from the tubing into the sheath. If the tubing has been poorly cleansed, this highly contaminated urine will then pool in the sheath and gain access to the urethra and eventually to the bladder. The tubing should be disinfected daily.

Collecting Bag or Jug: Allowing the collection bag or jug to overfill will prevent passage of urine away from the sheath and prevent the bladder from emptying properly (Fig. VII-1C). Poorly cleansed equipment will provide a source of bacterial contamination.

External catheters should be changed daily and usually are not suitable for reuse. Tubing, leg bags, night bottles or jugs can be reused but should be washed and disinfected daily (see Chap. XI, "Disinfection Procedures").

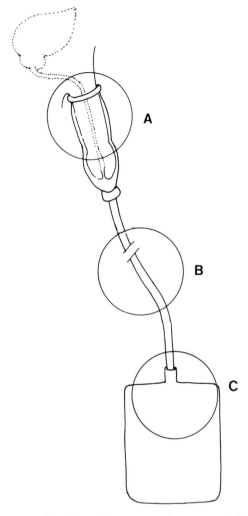

Figure VII-1. Danger areas where bacteria can enter the system. A. Perineal area and sheath. B. Tubing. C. Urine collecting bag or jug.

New tubing and urine collecting bags or jugs should be used weekly if financially feasible, with a maximum use of one month. If a patient is treated for a urinary tract infection, it is a good idea to replace all urinary equipment (i.e. tubing, leg bags, etc.) after taking an antibiotic for five to seven days to avoid reinfection from contaminated equipment.

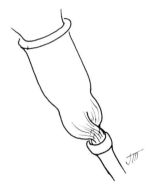

Figure VII-2. Twisting of external catheter obstructing urine flow.

Calculi

As with all patients with long-term urinary drainage problems, males using external catheters should be monitored closely for the formation of either renal or bladder calculi. Stones will form more readily in a concentrated alkaline urine. Frequently, patients using external catheters will cut down on their fluid intake to reduce the number of times it is necessary to "trigger" their bladder, or to minimize the number of times that their bladder empties spontaneously because they fear the external catheter might come off or leak. Consequently, it is necessary to reiterate the need for adequate fluid intake. See Chapters IV and XVII for more information regarding the formation and prevention of calculi.

Overdistention

Overdistention of the bladder wall can result in bladder sacules and diverticula, ureteral dilatation and back pressure to the kidneys. If bacteriuria exists, overdistention can lead to infection through microscopic breaks in the bladder lining and the rupture of capillaries in the bladder wall.

Overdistention can result when patients fail to trigger their bladder to empty at frequent intervals, when spontaneous voiding is disrupted or when sphincter dyssynergia occurs. If the external catheter or collecting appliance becomes twisted, kinked, or obstructed, urine flow from the bladder will be prevented and overdistention will develop.

Vesicoureteral Reflux

Vesicoureteral reflux, the passage of urine from the bladder through the ureters toward the kidneys, is another inherent danger for persons using external catheters. Infection and overdistention can damage the one-way valves that normally prevent the passage of urine from the bladder back up the ureter. Monitoring the urinary tract with periodic cystourethrograms will help identify the development of this problem before serious damage results. If bacteriuria is present, the passage of infected urine through the ureters and into the kidneys can lead to ureteritis and/or pyelonephritis. Even with sterile urine, the force of the urine back through the ureters into the kidneys can be sufficient to damage the renal parenchyma. This is sometimes referred to as the *water hammer effect.*

Mechanical Damage

Mechanical damage to the penis itself is always a major concern when using an external catheter. Extreme caution must be taken not to attach the appliance too tightly either with the adhesive tape provided or with additional tape. When a patient is first using an external catheter, it should be checked several times a day to ensure proper fit.[9] If the tape is on too tight, it can cut off circulation to the penis and/or prevent the flow of urine through the urethra. It can also result in tissue breakdown.

Occasionally, the rolled edge of the external catheter may be too tight and cut into the tissue. This can be alleviated by clipping the edge of the sheath after it is in place (Fig. VII-3).

Gentleness is essential when removing the external catheter. Careless pulling of the tape or adhesive can tear the tissue.

If irritation or sores develop on the shaft of the penis, replacement of the external catheter should be delayed for a period of time each day. If severe skin breakdown has occurred, it should be discontinued until the breakdown has healed. This may require temporary insertion of an indwelling catheter or changing to an intermittent catheterization program.

If the urine is alkaline, the head of the penis may become inflamed and irritated, particularly if the urine is allowed to pool in the appliance.

EFFECT OF DIET AND FLUID INTAKE

Accurate fluid intake and output records are an important aspect of patient care when one first begins using an external catheter. This will be of value in monitoring urine output and voiding patterns in relation to the amounts of fluid ingested.

Adequate fluid intake is essential to prevent renal and bladder calculi and to help wash out bacteria should infection occur. Consistent fluid intake, taken at frequent intervals, rather than drinking large amounts infrequently, will help to maintain and constantly dilute urine and regulate output.

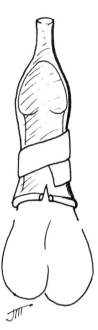

Figure VII-3. Rolled edge of external catheter clipped on underside to prevent tightness.

Unless medically countraindicated, fluid intake sufficient to provide an output of 2000 to 3000 ml per day is desirable. The best fluids to drink are water and cranberry juice (see Chap. V, "Effect of Diet and Fluid Intake").

Alcohol consumption should be avoided by all patients using external catheters. It will lead to tissue dehydration, which will affect urinary output, because the temporary increase in output will be followed by a decrease in output as body tissue fluids are replaced. This process will affect voiding schedules. Alcohol can affect the ability of the bladder wall to contract and lead to increased urinary residual and bladder overdistention. Alcohol has a dulling effect on the intellect which may lead patients to neglect to trigger their bladders to empty at the proper time, again leading to bladder overdistention and related problems. Severe overdistention in some spinal cord injured patients can result in autonomic dysreflexia which is potentially life threatening.

Diet plays an important part in the maintenance of acid urine. Certain foods produce a highly alkaline ash; these include foods high in citric acid such as oranges, tomatoes, and grapefruit. A list of foods contributing to alkaline urine is included in the Appendix.

Several medications have been suggested as good urine acidifiers. One is ascorbic acid (vitamin C) which is frequently given in doses of 500 mg four times a day. We have found that ascorbic acid is useful in keeping the urine acid, although some workers have had different results.[10] More carefully controlled research is needed to determine the effectiveness of this substance. Ascorbic acid should be used cautiously in stone formers, since some persons have defective metabolism of vitamin C resulting in increased urinary oxylate crystal formation.

Other medications suggested as urine acidifiers include Mandelamine® in large doses (approx. 2 grams, four times a day), methenamine hippurate and ammonium chloride. If ammonium chloride is used, serum levels of bicarbonate should be taken to establish the correct dosage and at periodic intervals thereafter to check for possible development of acidosis.

Excessive eating of high sodium foods will cause water retention with unpredictable diuresis (see Appendix, "Low Sodium Diet").

PHARMACOLOGICAL MANAGEMENT

We have indicated earlier that external drainage is used when bladder spasticity is forceful enough to open the bladder outlet or when sphincterotomy permits continuous outflow of urine. There are cases in which medications will allow the outlet to open in response to bladder contraction, although the timing of such activity cannot be controlled. A more extended discussion will be found in Chapter XIV, "Pharmacological Management of Bladder Kinetics." Briefly, the spastic internal sphincter will sometimes respond to phenoxybenzamine (Dibenzyline®) and a spastic external sphincter can sometimes be made less active by the use of muscle relaxants such as diazepam (Valium®), baclofen (Lioresal®) and dantroline (Dantrium®). All of these medications have side effects which can be harmful, requiring vigilance by both the patient and the health team. The functional effects should be monitored by residual urine measurement, cystometry and sometimes by urethral pressure profiles.

APPLIANCES

Types of External Catheters

There are several types of external catheters available. They are pictured in Figure VII-4.

Type A

This external catheter is made using a condom and a piece of tubing (Fig. VII-4A). The condom is stretched over the open end of the tubing and

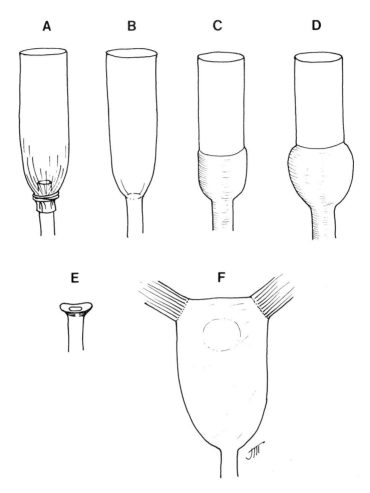

Figure VII-4. Types of external catheters. See text for description of each.

attached with a rubber band. A hole is cut in the condom so that urine can drain down the tubing. The condom is then secured on the shaft of the penis with skin adhesive or tape. Although this is a relatively inexpensive appliance, it has some distinct disadvantages. A condom is made of a very flexible material and easily twists, cutting off the flow of urine (Fig. VII-2). The inside of the condom must be handled when making the appliance, increasing the possibility of contamination with potentially pathogenic bacteria. This is particularly important if the condom becomes twisted, allowing urine to pool at the tip of the penis where the bacteria will multiply. When making the appliance, care must be taken to attach the condom close to the end of the tubing, because the tubing is frequently a firm plastic and the unprotected end inside the condom can be irritating to the skin. If skin bond is used to attach the condom, skin irritation may develop from the skin bond or the adhesive remover. If this occurs, it may be necessary to leave the external catheter off so that the skin can heal.

Type B

Type B is similar to type A except that it is obtained already assembled and individually packaged (Fig. VII-4B). It is made of condom-like material and a soft plastic tube. Because it is already assembled, there is less chance of gross contamination from handling. The sheath is flush with the tubing, with no rough sharp edges to irritate the glans. This type of external catheter has the disadvantage of twisting easily, allowing the urine to pool and preventing the bladder from emptying effectively. Type B external catheters are attached to the penis using skin bond or tape (example: Texas®).

Type C

There are several commercial products available similar to Type C (Fig. VII-4C). Essentially, they are all composed of a latex-type material which is heavier at the end joining the drainage tube. This helps to minimize the danger of twisting which leads to a pooling of urine and obstruction to outflow. Each comes packaged individually with some type of securing device (examples: Uro-san™ and Uri-Drain®).

A more recent product on the market has an adhesive material applied to the inside, eliminating the need for an adhesive strip. Patients with oily skin may find that this type of external catheter will not stay on (example: Freedom™).

Type D

External catheters similar to type D (Fig. VII-4D) are firmer than the type C sheaths, with the bulb and drainage tube being formed of an even more inflexible material. While there is no danger of twisting with this appliance, there is also minimal stretch so that there will be little expansion to accommodate an erection. Because of its size, shape and inflexibility, it is also more visible through clothing. The latex strap which is often supplied must be applied with care so that it will not constrict the penis (example: Uro® Sheath).

Type E

A relatively new external catheter consists of a short latex tube with a small bulge and flare at the end. The flare end is attached with adhesive directly to the end of the penis, with the opening to the tubing directly over the meatus (Fig. VII-4E). This appliance avoids covering the shaft of the penis and could be used by patients who develop skin abrasions or irritation from the condom-type external catheters. It has the disadvantage of being a little more difficult to apply. Sufficient adhesive must be applied to both the appliance and skin to obtain a good seal. A narrow strip of paper tape around the edge of the flared end will sometimes help keep the appliance in place (example: ARM 200 C Personal Care).

Type F

In addition to the above types of external catheters, there is another available that is essentially a urinal strapped over the penis. This may be a latex or rubber urinal with an opening through which the penis is inserted. It has an inner sheath which can be adjusted to fit the penis. The bag is then secured with a belt around the abdomen (Fig. VII-4F). A drainage tube in the lower end of the bag permits drainage into a collecting appliance. This type of external catheter has the advantage of not requiring attachment directly onto the skin of the penis. It has the disadvantage of being more expensive; however, it is reusable. It should be washed daily in order to keep clean and odor free. There may be leakage when the patient is lying down if the inner sheath does not fit snugly (example: McGuire Urinal®).

Undoubtedly, new products will continue to be developed and it is good to keep well informed of new appliances.

Type C and D come in different sizes. Using the best-fitting size will help eliminate some problems.

Methods of Securing External Catheters

Several types of adhesive materials can be used for securing the external catheter, and patients will frequently have to try several before finding the one that works best for them. Often, a combination of materials will be used.

Protective Dressing

A protective skin dressing is available that forms a clear barrier when used under an external catheter. It should be applied to the shaft of the penis after the skin has been washed and dried. The film is allowed to dry until it becomes tacky and then the external catheter applied. This protective skin dressing is available as individually packaged wipes, as a brush-on liquid or an aerosol. It is easily washed off with soap and water (example: Skin-Prep™).

Skin Adhesive

Skin adhesive is a bonding material that usually is obtained in a container with an application brush. The material is brushed onto the cleansed, dry skin on the shaft of the penis. After it dries to tackiness, the external catheter is rolled up over the bonding material and gently squeezed to seal. Skin adhesive, when properly applied, usually provides a moisture-proof seal. It is difficult and time-consuming to remove and requires use of an adhesive remover which is sometimes irritating to the skin (example: SkinBond®).[11]

Double-Faced Tape

There are at least two kinds of double-faced tape that come packaged with different type C external catheters. Each is about one inch wide and six inches long. One type is a sponge-like stretchy material; the other is a thin stretchy material. Either are applied to the clean dry skin on the penis (which may or may not have been treated with protective dressing). The tape is applied just behind the glans if the patient has been circumcised. If not circumcised, the foreskin *should not* be retracted but the tape applied about one-and-one-half inches from the tip of the penis. Apply the tape in a downward spiral fashion (towards the body) (Fig. VII-5A) with a slight overlapping. This allows for easier expansion if an erection occurs. The external catheter is then rolled up over the tape and gently squeezed to seal. External catheters attached in this manner can be removed by peeling back the catheter and tape.

Single-Faced Adhesive Tape

Some brands of external catheters, type C, are packaged with a foam tape that has adhesive material on only one side. This tape is applied *after* the appliance is in place on the penis. Starting about 1.5 inches from the tip of the penis and applying in a downward spiral (towards the body). To remove, peel off the tape and roll off the appliance (Fig. VII-5B).

Adhesive and Paper Tape

Frequently, patients will use ordinary waterproof adhesive tape or paper tape, either instead of or in addition to the adhesive stretchy tape.

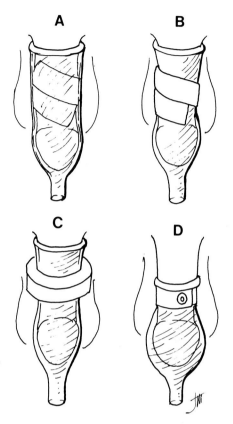

Figure VII-5. Methods for securing external catheter. A. Double-faced tape. B. Single-faced tape. C. Foam collar. D. Latex strap.

Extreme care must be taken to be sure the tape is not too tight, as this tape does not stretch. If this tape is applied directly to the skin, it may cause skin irritation.

Foam Collar

Some external catheters come with a foam rubber ring about one-quarter to one-half-inch thick and one-and-one-half to two inches in outside diameter (Fig. VII-4C). The inside hole will vary in size. The ring is stretched and slipped over the external catheter after it is in place. Care must be taken to be sure the ring is not too small leading to a *too tight* fit which may cause skin erosion and/or cut off circulation. To remove, slide off the foam collar and roll off the appliance (example: Davol™).

Straps

A latex strap is usually supplied with a type D external catheter. It must be applied with care so that it will not be too tight (Fig. VII-5D).

Commercially prepared external catheter straps are available consisting of a foam strip with an elastic band and Velcro® closure (e.g. Condom Catheter Holder, BeOk, Fred Sammons Inc.). These straps can be wrapped around the outside of the condom to secure it. Care must be taken not to attach it too tight. A loop placed at the end of the strip will aid persons with limited dexterity (Fig. VII-6).

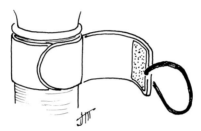

Figure VII-6. Foam strap (e.g. Condom Catheter Holder, BeOK—Fred Sammons Inc.) with a loop attached to facilitate use.

Urine Collection Appliances

The external catheter is attached to a tubing either directly or with an adapter. The tubing is then connected to a urine collection receptacle. Clear plastic tubing is recommended because the condition of the inside of the tubing is more readily visible and because the smooth inside surface helps reduce the buildup of extraneous material and bacterial growth. For daytime use the tubing can be relatively short and attached to a leg bag (Fig. VII-7). For night or in bed the tubing should be long enough to permit movement and be attached to a bag, jug or bottle. See Chapter V "Open Drainage System" for a detailed description.

CARE PROCEDURES

Wash hands vigorously before working with urinary appliances to minimize the chance of contamination. Although patients caring for themselves usually do not wear gloves, it is recommended that all others wear nonsterile gloves to protect their hands from infection. This is particularly important with the increase in urogenital diseases such as *herpes.*

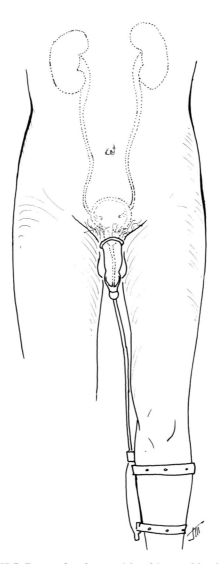

Figure VII-7. External catheter with tubing and leg bag attached.

Wash the perineal area and penis with a mild detergent, retracting the foreskin if not circumcised. Dry skin well and check for skin abrasions. Push back pubic hair to avoid catching it in condom or tape. Occasionally, it may be necessary to shave off excessive hair. (Be sure to replace foreskin.)

If a skin adhesive is used, apply evenly over entire length of penis except for the glans and allow to dry until it becomes tacky. Apply the external catheter using the procedure appropriate for the type used (see "Types of External Catheters").

Some patients feel more secure if they apply additional tape after the appliance is in place. Care must be taken not to apply this tape too tightly.

Attach tubing to appliance to drain the urine into a leg bag, night bag or jug. Avoid twists in the tubing and appliance which could cut off urine flow. Sometimes, it is necessary to use an adapter between the appliance and tubing to prevent twisting and to facilitate connection (Fig. VII-8).

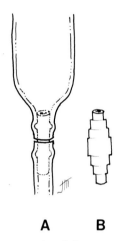

A   B

Figure VII-8. A. A straight connector placed between an external catheter and tubing. B. A Christmas tree (5-in-1) connector which could also be used to connect an external catheter to tubing.

If a leg bag is used, the straps should always be placed through the leg bag in such a way that they lie behind the bag (see Chap. XI, "Positioning Urinary Drainage Equipment"). If the straps are placed so they are in front of the main section of the bag, they will tighten as the bag fills, hindering circulation and causing swelling of the foot.

Appliance Care

As already stated, the external catheter should be changed daily. The tubing, leg bag and night drainage system should be washed and disinfected daily to prevent a build up of bacteria that could lead to urinary tract infections (see Chap. XI, "Disinfection Procedures").

IMPORTANT THINGS TO REMEMBER ABOUT EXTERNAL CATHETERS

1. Always wash hands well before and after urinary drainage appliance care. *Put on non-sterile gloves.*
2. Before applying external catheter, wash genital area, retracting fore-

skin if patient is not circumcised. Thoroughly cleanse area around glans. Dry area well and replace foreskin.

3. Remove excessive hair in pubic area.

4. Check penis for abrasions or redness and report any to the physician.

5. Follow instructions for specific external catheter being used. Application instructions vary with different products.

6. Change external catheter every 24 hours.

7. Always place drainage tubing in descending line from bladder to urine collecting device.

8. Be sure the tubing connecting external catheter to leg bag is correct length so it does not twist, loop or pull too tight when leg is outstretched.

9. Use new sterile or disinfected drainage equipment daily (tubing, leg bag, night bag or jug).

10. Encourage consistent fluid intake and regular bladder emptying if bladder can be triggered to empty or emptied at will.

E.N.

REFERENCES

1. Hull, M.H.: Appliances for the incontinent patient. *Brit J Urol 37*:644–649, 1965.
2. Lawson, S.D., and Cook, J.B.: Condom urinals. *Nurs Mirror 145*:19–21, Dec. 1, 1977.
3. Golji, H.: Urethral sphincterotomy for chronic spinal cord injury. *J Urol 123*:204–7, 1980.
4. Van-Arsdalen, K.N., Klein, F.A., Hackler, R.H., and Brady, S.M.: Penile implants in spinal cord injury patients for maintaining external appliances. *J Urol 126*:331–332, 1981.
5. Smith, A.D., Sazama, R., and Lange, P.H.: Penile prosthesis: Adjunct to treatment of patients with neurogenic bladder. *J Urol 124*:363–364, 1980.
6. Newman, E., and Price, M.: Bacteriuria in patients with spinal cord lesions: Its relationship to urinary drainage appliances. *Arch Phys Med Rehabil 58*:427–430, 1978.
7. Hinman, F., and Cox, C.E.: The voiding vesical defense mechanism: The mathematical effect of residual urine, voiding interval and volume on bacteruria. *J Urol 96*:491–498, 1966.
8. Merritt, J.L.: Residual urine volume: Correlate of urinary tract infection in patients with spinal cord injury. *Arch Phys Med Rehab 62*:558–561, 1981.
9. Golji, H.: Complications of external condom drainage. *Paraplegia 19*:189–197, 1981.
10. Devenport, J.K., Swenson, J.R., Dukes, G.E., and Sonsalla, P.K. Formaldehyde generation from methenamine salts in spinal cord injury. *Arch Phys Med Rehabil 65*:257–259, 1984.
11. Bransbury, A.J.: Allergy to rubber condom urinals and medical adhesives in male spinal cord injury patients. *Contact Dermatitis 5*:317–323, 1979.

Chapter VIII

INTERMITTENT CATHETERIZATION

I ntermittent catheterization is a method of urinary drainage that involves the periodic catheterization of the bladder to drain the urine. This method of urinary management has been used with varying degrees of success since World War I. Sir Ludvig Guttman[1] began using intermittent catheterization on a large scale for patients with spinal cord injury during World War II. Although he reported excellent results, the method did not acquire widespread use because of the necessity of trained personnel to perform the required catheterization and because of concern regarding the long-term affect of multiple catheterizations on the integrity of the urethra.

In more recent years there has been a renewed interest in intermittent catheterization because it resembles the normal process of filling and emptying. There has been no definitive evidence reported that repeated urethral catheterization leads to urethral trauma. However, the need for adequately trained personnel remains.

INDICATIONS FOR USE

Intermittent catheterization may be considered whenever there is a condition affecting the normal process of micturition provided there are not other contraindications such as urethral strictures or trauma.

Intermittent catheterization is frequently used for the patient with a neurogenic bladder, that is, when bladder function has been modified by some interference with the nerve supply. If the neurogenic bladder develops as the result of trauma to the spinal cord, the bladder may remain in a state of spinal shock for a varying period of time. It is during this period that some investigators[1,2] feel intermittent catheterization mimicking the normal filling and emptying of the bladder will result in a more rapid recovery of detrusor reflex activity. This phase of bladder management is usually carried out in an acute care, rehabilitation or extended care facility where there is sufficient trained personnel. If reflex voiding has not returned by the time the patient is discharged from these facilities, the intermittent catheterization program may or may not be continued, depending in part upon the patient's ability to self-catheterize or the availability of assistance.

Intermittent catheterization programs are also being used for persons with meningomyelocele or spina bifida, conditions which previously frequently resulted in urinary diversion.[3] Intermittent catheterization is also often used for patients who experience a temporary loss of ability to void on command due to surgery, childbirth or an episode of severe overdistention.

INHERENT DANGERS

The dangers of intermittent catheterization are related to four general conditions: *bacteriuria, bladder overdistention, urethral trauma* and *calculi.* Problems which may develop as the result of these four conditions include invasive urinary tract infection, septicemia, reflux, hydronephrosis, epididymitis, urethral stricture and urethral diverticula.

The incidence of bacteriuria in patients using intermittent catheterization, while much lower than for patients with indwelling catheters, is still high.[4] In our patients, bacteriuria was found in over 50 percent. Bacteriuria accompanied by overdistention can lead to bacterial tissue invasion with resultant bladder wall infection and the potential for kidney infection, septicemia and/or epididymitis. Infection is thought to be spread by both vascular and lymphatic vessels. Repeated overdistention and infection can lead to scarring and thickening of the bladder wall with the development of bladder trabeculations, saccules, diverticula and reflux. The irregularities produced in the bladder wall permit "pooling" of urine which reduces the efficiency of bladder washout, increasing the potential for infection and calculus formation.

The risk of urethral irritation does not appear to be as great as previously anticipated provided there is no pre-existing urethral stricture or diverticulum. Care must be taken to lubricate the catheter adequately and to avoid excessive force when passing the catheter.

The potential for calculus formation is reduced in patients on intermittent catheterization as opposed to those on indwelling catheters by virtue of the absence of a foreign body within the bladder. However, the maintenance of dilute acidic urine is still recommended to further reduce the danger of calculus formation, particularly in a newly immobilized person.

EFFECT OF DIET AND FLUID INTAKE

Diet

As with all patients with long-term urinary drainage problems, an effort should be made to keep the urine acid. Many bacteria causing urinary tract infections will grow best in a neutral or alkaline medium. Calcium will also remain in solution better in acid urine, thereby reducing the danger of bladder or renal calculi. Some foods when consumed produce an alkaline ash which increases the urinary pH. Perhaps the worst offenders in this matter are the citrus fruits. This would seem contradictory since these foods are high in vitamin C, a substance frequently given in an attempt to acidify the urine. However, other components such as citric acid contribute to an alkaline ash which offsets the acidifying effect of the vitamin C present. Foods producing acid and alkaline ash are listed in the Appendix.

Fluid Intake

Careful monitoring of fluid intake is important when establishing an intermittent catheterization program, as the frequency of bladder catheterization will be influenced by the amount and regularity of fluid intake. Generally, a fluid intake of 2500 ml with even distribution throughout the day is recommended. The best fluids to drink are water and cranberry juice, particularly if the patient is having problems with urinary tract infections, as most other fluids (e.g. orange juice, soda pop and fruit drinks) tend to alkalinize the urine.

Alcoholic beverages should be avoided for several reasons. First, alcohol affects urinary output. Alcohol consumption will result in tissue dehydration and a temporary increase in urinary output, followed by a period of decreased urinary output as the tissue fluids are replaced. This temporary irregularity in output will affect the urine volumes and require adjustments in catheterization schedules to avoid overdistention. Second, alcohol affects the contractability of the bladder wall, thus affecting the ability of the bladder to empty spontaneously. Third, alcohol consumption has a dulling effect on the intellect which may cause patients to forget or disregard the need for catheterization resulting in bladder overdistention.

Dairy products are frequently limited for patients with long-term urinary problems to decrease urinary calcium excretion, lowering the risk of bladder or kidney calculi.

CATHETERIZATION SCHEDULE

The object of intermittent catheterization is to allow the bladder to fill and empty in a manner that mimics normal function; however, it is extremely important that the bladder not be allowed to become overdistended. This is particularly important for a patient where a return of detrusor contraction is anticipated. Therefore, accurate records of intake and output are essential to establish a urinary output pattern. Generally, with a daily output of 1500 to 2000 ml, catheterization every four hours is adequate. If the volume of urine obtained with a catheterization exceeds 400 ml, catheterization should be increased to every three hours, or even more frequently, to maintain volumes at each catheterization below 400 ml.

Careful record keeping of input and output as well as time of catheterization will help establish a pattern. Once the protocol is established, it is important to maintain a consistent fluid intake and to be aware of the need to adjust the catheterization schedule if there has been a marked deviation from routine fluid intake. Ingestion of diuretics or water-retaining foods, dependent edema or night diuresis will also affect output and may require adjustment of catheterization schedule. For some patients who have large nocturnal volumes, especially patients over 60 years of age, it may be necessary to limit fluid intake after 10 P.M.

PHARMACOLOGICAL MANAGEMENT

Sometimes, problems with incontinence between catheterization can be managed pharmacologically. Incontinence due to bladder wall spasticity can often be lessened by anticholinergic drugs such as methanetheline (Banthine®), propantheline (Pro-Banthine®) or oxybutynin (Ditropan®). See Chapter XIV "Pharmacological Control of Bladder Kinetics" for more information.

DAILY CARE—CATHETERIZATION PROCEDURES

After careful record keeping of intake and output, work out the catheterization schedule that is best for each individual.

Choose a catheterizing procedure that presents the least risk of infection and yet meets the financial needs of the patient.

There is considerable difference of opinion regarding the use of sterile or non-sterile catheterization procedures for intermittent catheterization programs. It is generally accepted, though, that sterile technique is a must in the acute phase in all health care facilities to minimize the danger of nosocomial infections with potentially pathogenic organisms.[2] However, for post-discharge care some physicians will recommend a clean catheterization program.

Regardless of the method of catheterization used, it is important to prevent damage to the bladder mucosa and renal parenchyma. Increased intravesical pressure and/or bladder overdistention can produce a decrease in blood flow. The ischemic bladder will be susceptible to bacterial invasion.[5] *Close adherence to a catheterization schedule that will prevent overdistention is imperative.*

Some health care facilities have developed catheterization teams that do all the catheterization. In other instances, catheterization is performed by allied health care personnel, while frequently patients are taught to catheterize themselves.

Perineal Care

The perineal area and meatus should be carefully cleaned with detergent and water and/or povidone-iodine solution before each catheterization.

Sterile Intermittent Catheterization

Many facilities have established catheterization protocols. A "no-touch" sterile catheterization procedure can be found in Chapter V. By substituting a simple sterile Robinson catheter for the Foley catheter, this method may be used for intermittent catheterization.

Recently, several catheters have been developed especially for intermittent catheterization. One such catheter[6] comes packaged within a plastic pouch that has a protected top chamber through which the catheter is passed The penis is carefully cleaned with povidone-iodine solution. The top chamber which consists of a rigid collar is opened and lubricant added. The collar is then placed directly over the glans penis and the catheter is fed through the lubricant into the urethra and bladder. The urine flows out through the catheter into the pouch. When the bladder is empty, the catheter is withdrawn, the urine observed for volume and discarded. (e.g. Bard® Touchless®)

There is also a catheter adapted for females with a slightly different top chamber. Both types require practice to develop efficiency, but many patients learn self-catheterization quite readily with these catheters.

Care must be taken when using this type of catheter to carefully cleanse the penis and meatus before passing the catheter and to avoid missing the meatus and sliding the catheter along the side of the penis resulting in contamination. This catheter has the advantage of being entirely enclosed up to the point of insertion eliminating several possibilities of contamination. It does not allow for a great deal of flexibility of movement and this may make insertion more difficult for some patients.

Also available are individually packaged sterile catheters for self-catheterization that are made of a transparent plastic-type material. They are available from several manufacturers in male, female and pediatric sizes. They may be used in place of the red rubber catheter for sterile no-touch technique and are sometimes used for at-home catheterization. They are less flexible than the red rubber catheter and care must be taken to avoid urethral trauma.

Non-Sterile Catheterization

Cost becomes a major factor when considering a long-term program of intermittent catheterization (e.g., catheter kits at $4.50 × 6 cath/day = $27.00/day). Partly because of the cost, some physicians have permitted the use of a modified "sterile" procedure after discharge from the health care facility. The risk of infection and the cost of antibiotics if infection occurs, as well as other conditions, must be carefully weighed against the cost of supplies when planning an intermittent catheterization program.

The following procedure allows for the disinfection and reuse of the catheter and the use of individually packaged products rather than trays or kits.

If it is necessary to reuse catheters, they should be carefully cleansed and disinfected. The method of disinfection used will depend upon the type of catheter. The clear plastic-type catheters are best disinfected by alcohol, as boiling will make them cloudy and brittle. The red rubber (Robinson) type of catheter may be disinfected by boiling or a combination of boiling and alcohol.

Modifications of these semi-sterile catheterization procedures are occasionally made by physician, health care professionals or patients. For example, non-sterile gloves may be substituted for sterile gloves. Povidone-iodine solution and rayon balls may be substituted for swabs or wipes. It is important to remember that each departure from sterile supplies and techniques increases the chance of infection and this risk should be carefully considered when designing a protocol for a patient.

Male Catheterization with Reusable Catheter

The following protocols are designed for male *self-catheterization* but can be adapted for assisted catheterization.

Supplies Needed

- Sterile, individually packaged straight catheter.
- Povidone-iodine swabs or wipes or povidone-iodine solution and rayon balls.
- Sterile gauze squares individually packaged.
- Lubricating jelly, tube or individual packages.
- Gloves, sterile or non-sterile. If non-sterile gloves are used, do not use

the same box used for bowel program. Do not completely remove cover but open partially so box remains covered when not in use. Be careful not to contaminate gloves. Treat as sterile gloves.
- Denatured 70 percent alcohol plus container and cover to hold catheter and alcohol. Use ethyl, propyl or isopropyl (70% rubbing alcohol), not methyl.
- Waterproof pad or towel.
- Detergent and water.
- Receptacle.

Procedure with New Catheter (Male):

1. Obtain necessary supplies.
2. Wash hands.
3. Place waterproof pad or towel on knees and position receptacle.
4. Wash perineal area.
5. Clean penis with povidone-iodine solution; retract foreskin if not circumcised. If the patient is allergic to povidone-iodine, cleanse well with a detergent and water.
6. Open catheter (peel back paper while it is lying on knees).
7. Lubricate catheter (if using tube, discard first $1/2$ inch of lubricant). Squeeze lubricant onto catheter.
8. Put on gloves.
9. Pick up catheter with dominant hand (avoid touching the tip of the catheter).
10. Hold penis with non-dominant hand and pass catheter through meatus into bladder.
11. Drain urine into receptacle. Be sure to empty bladder well. Use light pressure on abdomen.
12. Remove catheter.
13. Wash penis to remove povidone-iodine and lubricant.
14. Reposition foreskin if not circumcised.
15. Wipe lubricant from catheter. Wash catheter well with detergent inside and out. Be sure all lubricant is removed. Rinse and dry catheter.
16. Disinfect catheter (see "Disinfection of Catheters for Reuse.")

Procedure with Reused Catheter (Male)

1. Obtain supplies.
2. Wash hands.
3. Place waterproof pad or towel on knees and position receptacle.

4. Wash perineal area, retract foreskin if not circumcised.
5. Cleanse penis with povidone-iodine. If the patient is allergic to povidone-iodine, cleanse well with a detergent and water.
6. Open sterile gauze package, peel back paper and lay package on knees.
7. Place lubricant on sterile gauze (discard first 1/2 inch from tube).
8. Put on gloves.
9. Remove catheter from alcohol. Allow it to drain and drip dry. You may wipe catheter dry with sterile gauze square. There are usually two gauze squares in the package. One may be used to wipe the catheter dry of alcohol and the other used for lubricant.
10. Pick up sterile gauze on which lubricant has been placed and lubricate catheter.
11. Hold penis with non-dominant hand and pass catheter through meatus into bladder. Drain urine into receptacle. Be sure to empty bladder well. Use light pressure on abdomen.
12. Remove catheter and wash self. Replace foreskin if not circumcised.
13. Wipe lubricant off catheter.
14. Wash catheter well inside and out in detergent. Be sure all lubricant is washed off. Rinse and dry catheter.
15. Disinfect catheters (see "Disinfection of Catheters for Reuse").

If using the clear plastic type catheter, it is recommended that a new sterile catheter be used each A.M., reused after disinfection for catheterizations during that day, and then discarded.

Alcohol should be discarded and replaced with new fresh alcohol at least once a week. Alcohol should be kept in a covered container to avoid evaporation.

Ambulatory male patients may find they are able to catheterize in a standing position, in which case they will need a convenient area where supplies can be laid out.

Female Self-Catheterization with a Reusable Catheter

Female self-catheterization is more difficult, particularly if the patient is not ambulatory, as it will require transfer to a bed. Ambulatory patients can frequently work out a procedure whereby they stand with one foot elevated to better expose the perineal area. If self-catheterizing is done in a supine position, a mirror is often necessary for better viewing the site of insertion.

Supplies Needed

- Sterile, individually packaged straight catheter.
- Povidone-iodine swabs or wipes.
- Sterile gauze squares individually packaged.
- Lubricating jelly, tube or individual packages.
- Gloves—sterile or non-sterile. If non-sterile gloves are used, do not use the same box used for bowel program. Do not completely open cover. Open partially so box remains covered when not in use. Be careful not to contaminate gloves. Treat as sterile gloves.
- Seventy percent alcohol plus container and cover to hold catheter and alcohol. Use ethyl, isopropyl (70% rubbing alcohol), not methyl.
- Waterproof pad or towel.
- Detergent and water.
- Mirror.
- Forceps.

Procedure with New Catheter—Supine Position (Female)

1. Obtain necessary supplies and place in convenient position.
2. Wash hands.
3. Open catheter—peel back paper and leave catheter lying on paper.
4. Lubricate catheter (if using tube, discard first 1/2 inch).
5. Place waterproof pad on bed.
6. Assume supine position, spreading knees apart.
7. Wash perineal area.
8. Cleanse all parts of perineum with povidone-iodine solution. Leave last swab or wipe between labia. If patient is allergic to povidone-iodine, cleanse well with a detergent and water.
9. Place receptacle in convenient location.
10. Put on gloves.
11. With dominant hand, pick up catheter.
12. With other hand, remove povidone-iodine swab and hold labia apart.
13. Pass catheter into bladder. Some patients learn to feel the meatus with non-dominant hand, while others may use a mirror. If mirror is used, it should be positioned before putting on gloves.
14. Drain urine into receptacle. Be sure to empty bladder completely. Use slight pressure on abdomen.
15. Remove catheter.
16. Wash self.
17. Wipe lubricant from catheter.

18. Wash catheter inside and out with detergent. Be sure all lubricant is removed. Rinse and dry.
19. Disinfect catheters (see "Disinfection of Catheters for Reuse").

Procedure with Reused Catheter Supine Position (Female)

1. Obtain necessary supplies.
2. Wash hands.
3. Peel open sterile package. Allow wrapper to serve as sterile field.
4. Place lubricant on sterile gauze (if using tube, discard first one-half inch of lubricant).
5. With forcep, remove catheter from alcohol, drain and lay on sterile field. Pick up catheter by flared end to avoid contamination of tip.
6. Place waterproof pad on bed.
7. Assume supine position and place receptacle in a convenient place.
8. Wash perineal area, separating labia.
9. Cleanse all parts of the perineum with povidone-iodine. Leave last swab or wipe between labia. If the patient is allergic to povidone-iodine, cleanse well with detergent and water.
10. Put on gloves.
11. Pick up catheter with dominant hand.
12. With other hand, remove povidone-iodine swab or wipe and hold labia apart.
13. Pass catheter into bladder and drain urine. Some patients learn to find site with non-dominant hand; others may use mirror. If a mirror is used, it should be positioned before putting on gloves.
14. Be sure to empty bladder completely. Use light abdominal pressure.
15. Remove catheter.
16. Wash self.
17. Wash catheter with detergent, rinse, and dry.
18. Disinfect catheter (see "Disinfection of Catheters for Reuse").
19. If a clear plastic type catheter is used, take a new catheter for first catheterization each day. Reuse after disinfection for that day only, because build up of lubricant will reduce effectiveness of disinfectant.

Disinfection of Catheters for Reuse

Clear Plastic Catheters (e.g. Self-Cath™)

It is recommended that a *new sterile* catheter be used each morning. The catheter can then be disinfected with alcohol for reuse that day. A new *sterile* catheter should be used the next morning. Using a new sterile catheter each day is necessary because the lubricant will gradually collect on and in the catheter with repeated use (even with washing), making the alcohol disinfection less effective.

Procedure: Alcohol Disinfection Clear Plastic Catheter

1. Wipe off lubricant.
2. Wash catheter with a *detergent* (e.g. Dreft®) and water inside and outside. Use a catheter-tipped syringe or squirt bottle to force the solution through the catheter. Check catheter to be sure all lubricant has been removed. Do not wash with a *soap,* as this will leave film on the catheter.
3. Rinse and dry. Be sure water is out of tip of catheter. Water left in the catheter will dilute the alcohol.
4. Place catheter in a covered container of 70 percent ethyl or isopropyl alcohol (rubbing alcohol). Be sure alcohol fills the catheter and that catheter is covered with alcohol.
5. Leave catheters in alcohol for *at least 10 minutes* or until next use.
6. To reuse, remove catheter from the alcohol. Drain to dry before reuse. Be careful not to contaminate the catheter.

The alcohol container should be covered to prevent evaporation. The alcohol should be discarded and replaced with fresh alcohol once a week.

More than one *clean* catheter can be placed in alcohol at one time. Be sure all of them fill with alcohol and are completely covered with it. This will require a larger container and larger amount of alcohol (more expense) than if only one catheter is disinfected at a time. If you are going to be away from home, you may find it more convenient to put an *alcohol disinfected* catheter in a new Ziploc type plastic bag with a small amount of alcohol. The used catheter can be returned to the bag for storage until you are home again, where it can be cleaned and disinfected. DO NOT REUSE THIS BAG FOR A DISINFECTED CATHETER.

Disinfection of Red Rubber (Robinson) Catheters

Red rubber (Robinson) catheters can be disinfected with alcohol provided they are free of all lubricant. Because it is impossible to see inside the rubber catheters to determine if all lubricant has been removed, it is recommended that all used catheters be boiled to free them from lubricant before alcohol disinfection.

You may wish to boil a number of catheters at a time, dry and store them for reuse with alcohol disinfection.

Procedure: Disinfection of Red Rubber Catheters with Alcohol

1. Place *clean* (boiled) catheter in a covered container of 70 percent ethyl or isopropyl alcohol (rubbing alcohol). Be sure catheter fills with alcohol and is completely covered.
2. Leave catheter in alcohol until ready to use (for at least 10 minutes).
3. To use catheter, remove from alcohol and allow to drain dry. Do not contaminate catheter.
4. Catheterize self. See procedure.
5. Place another *clean* catheter in the alcohol for next catheterization.

The alcohol container should be covered to prevent evaporation. The alcohol should be discarded and replaced with fresh alcohol once a week.

Procedure for Boiling Red Rubber (Robinson) Catheters

1. Before boiling, all catheters should be wiped free of lubricant, washed with a detergent and water solution. Flush solution through catheter using a catheter-tipped syringe or squirt bottle. Rinse well.
2. Place catheters in a kettle of water. Cover and bring to a boil. Be sure to use enough water so the kettle does not boil dry.
3. Boil 30 minutes. (It is not necessary to boil vigorously; you may turn down the heat so water is just boiling.)
4. Remove from heat. Catheters are now disinfected and how you handle them now will depend on how and when you plan to use the catheters.
   a. If you have boiled a number of catheters and plan to place them in alcohol for 10 minutes before use, drain dry and store them in a covered container. They are now ready to be placed in alcohol for at least 10 minutes before use.
   b. If you plan to use the boiled catheters without alcohol disinfection, you must be careful not to contaminate the catheters. Drain the catheters and allow them to dry. Tip the kettle from side to side to allow water to drain out of catheters. If you drain them while the water is hot, they tend to dry faster; however, extreme care must be taken to avoid burning yourself. The dry catheters can be stored in a sterile covered jar (boil jar and cover 30 minutes to sterilize) or placed in *new* plastic bags (Ziploc™ type sandwich bags work well). Store only *one* catheter in a bag to avoid contamination of others when removing one for use. Use a disinfected forceps to transfer the catheters. Do not touch catheters with your hands. Be careful not to contaminate catheters. *Do not reuse the bags.*

Several days' supply of used catheters may be boiled at one time, allowed to dry and stored for future alcohol disinfection and use. It is recommended, however, that the catheter used each day be wiped free of lubricant, washed in detergent and rinsed before being saved for future boiling.

Disinfection of Forceps or Clamp: Place forceps in alcohol for 10 minutes or boil for 30 minutes. Boiling can be accomplished by hanging the forceps from edge of container into water while boiling the catheters.

IMPORTANT THINGS TO REMEMBER
ABOUT INTERMITTENT CATHETERIZATION

1. Maintain consistent fluid intake to help regulate catheterization schedule. Avoid alcohol consumption.
2. Maintain an acid urine.
3. Catheterize at scheduled times. Do not permit bladder overdistention. It is better to catheterize sooner than necessary than later.
4. Wash hands before beginning catheterization.
5. Cleanse perineal area with povidone-iodine or detergent and water before catheterizing.
6. Be sure to lubricate catheter well to avoid urethral irritation.
7. It is recommended that sterile catheterization procedures be used in all health care facilities. For "at home" catheterization, maintain as near a sterile procedure as possible. Remember that each departure from sterile technique increases the risk of infection.
8. Be aware of the signs and symptoms of a urinary tract infection. Report their occurrence to the physicians.

E.N.

REFERENCES

1. Guttman, L., and Frankel, H.: The value of intermittent catheterization in the early management of traumatic paraplegia and tetraplegia. *Paraplegia 4:*63–84, 1966.
2. Comarr, A.E.: Intermittent catheterization for the traumatic cord bladder patient. *J Urol 108:*79–81, 1972.
3. Drago, J.R., Wellner, L., Sanford, E.J., and Rohner, T.J., Jr.: The role of intermittent catheterization in the management of children with myelomeningocele. *J Urol 118:*92–94, 1977.
4. Erickson, R.P., Merritt, J.L., Opitz, J.L., and Ilstrup, D.M.: Bacteriuria during follow-up in patients with spinal cord injury: 1. Rates of bacteriuria in various bladder-emptying methods. *Arch Phys Med Rehabil 63:*409–412, 1982.
5. Lapides, J., Diokno, A.C., Silber, S.J. and Lowe, B.S.: Clean, intermittent self-catheterization in the treatment of urinary tract disease. *J Urol 107:*458–461, 1972.
6. Wu, Y., King, R.B., Hamilton, B.B., and Betts, H.B.: RIC–Wu catheter kit: New device for an old problem. *Arch Phys Med Rehabil 61:*455–459, 1980.

Chapter IX

APPLIANCE-FREE STATE

The term *appliance-free voiding* implies that no urinary drainage appliances are required. Three conditions are necessary for the appliance-free state. First, voiding must occur on command, either spontaneously or when triggered. Second, the bladder must empty adequately with voiding. Third, the patient must remain manageably continent between voidings.

INDICATIONS FOR USE

Some patients with the potential for long-term urinary problems can avoid using urinary drainage appliances and, with careful management, remain appliance free. Other patients who have experienced conditions such as trauma, surgery or diseases initially requiring the use of artificial urinary drainage may eventually regain the appliance-free state. This is often accomplished through a program of *bladder training*[1] or *trial off catheter.* (A trial off catheter protocol is included in the Appendix.) The number of patients attaining the catheter-free state is increasing as patients and health care professionals learn more about urinary tract management.

Occasionally, although desirable in terms of prevention of renal deterioration, the appliance-free state is impractical. For example, a spinal cord injured person may be continent and able to trigger voiding but require assistance to transfer to a toilet, remove clothing or to place a receptacle, greatly limiting independence and perhaps requiring full-time attendant care. Or, a person may spend his/her day in an environment (e.g. school or work place) where facilities are not readily available, leading to infrequent voiding with bladder overdistention and/or incontinence. The practicality of the appliance-free state must be carefully weighed against the long-term health benefits.

INHERENT DANGERS

Although appliance-free voiding is a non-invasive method of drainage, the potential for long-term problems still remain and careful monitoring to identify and prevent them is important.[2]

144

Two conditions most frequently resulting in urinary tract complications are infection and bladder overdistention.

Infection

We have found that about one-third of our spinal cord injured patients, who have attained the appliance-free state, have positive urine cultures when they return for their annual renal function evaluations.[3] A high incidence of bacteriuria in populations of appliance-free geriatric patients has also been reported.[4]

Several reasons can be suggested for the high rate of bacteriuria. First, prior to attaining the catheter-free state, the patients may have developed a deep-seated urinary tract infection which periodically flares up. Second, infrequent and incomplete bladder emptying may prevent the normal "bladder washout" of bacteria that migrate into the bladder through the urethra. Third, bladder overdistention and infection may lead to the development of bladder trabeculation and diverticula. Urine pooling in these bladder wall irregularities becomes stagnant, reducing the effectiveness of bladder washout.

Infection may be confined to the bladder or bacteria may reach the kidney and result in pyelonephritis.

Overdistention

Bladder overdistention and infection may lead to diverticula, or saccule formation, and perpetuate bacteriuria as discussed above. It may also result in the development of vesicoureteral reflux, the backflow of urine towards the kidneys. In addition to carrying bacteria into the kidney, reflux can result in renal parenchyma damage from the actual force of the urine against the tissue. This is referred to as the water hammer effect.

Chronic overdistention will weaken the bladder and ureteral walls preventing the entire system from emptying adequately, leading to increased pressure and the development of hydronephrosis.

Calculi

Although the incidence of bladder and/or renal calculi in patients who have attained the appliance-free state is lower than in patients with other methods of urinary drainage, the potential for developing calculi remains. This potential is directly proportional to the incidence of infection, stagnant and alkaline urine.

EFFECT OF DIET AND FLUID INTAKE

Frequently, patients who are appliance free will limit their fluid intake to reduce the need for bladder emptying or to minimize the danger of incontinence. However, a good *consistent* fluid intake is important to reduce the dangers of infection and/or calculi formation. Intake sufficient to maintain an output of approximately 2000 ml per day is recommended unless medically contraindicated.

As with all methods of urinary drainage, urine acidification will help prevent bacteriuria and calculi formation. Good fluids to drink are water and cranberry juice (see Chap. V, "The Effect of Diet and Fluid Intake").

Alcohol should be avoided for several reasons but particularly because of its inhibiting effect on the contraction of the bladder wall leading to overdistention and increased urinary residual (see Chap. VII, "The Effect of Diet and Fluid Intake").

Diet plays an important role in the maintenance of acid urine. A list of foods contributing to urine alkalinization is included in the Appendix. Notable among the foods to avoid are those high in citric acid, such as oranges, lemons and tomatoes. These foods should be avoided if the person is experiencing frequent urinary tract infections and/or calculi.

Several medications have been suggested as urine acidifiers. Ascorbic acid (vitamin C), Mandelamine, Hiprex® and ammonium chloride have all been reported with varying degrees of success. There is a need for carefully controlled research in this area.

PHARMACOLOGICAL MANAGEMENT

Spontaneous and controlled emptying of the bladder may develop from increasing awareness of bladder fullness or from reinnervation of a defectively innervated bladder. On the other hand, partially innervated bladders can sometimes achieve almost normal function without these developments by means of medication. This subject is treated more fully in Chapter XIII, "Pharmacological Control of Bladder Kinetics." In brief, bladder wall spasticity can often be lessened by anticholinergic drugs such as methantheline (Banthine), propantheline (Pro-banthine®) or oxybutynin (Ditropan), while weak bladder contractions can frequently be strengthened by the cholinergic bethanacol (Urecholine®, Duvoid®). Internal sphincter spasticity can sometimes be modulated by phenoxybenzamine (Dibenzyline) and external sphincter spasticity by muscle relaxants such as diazepam (Valium), baclofen (Lioresal), and dantrolene (Dantrium). All medications have potentially dangerous side effects, for which users and prescribers must be vigilant. The effectiveness of bladder-controlling drugs must be monitored by periodic residual urine measurements as well as by the use of cystometry.

MONITORING AND FOLLOW-UP CARE

Patients who are at risk for urinary tract pathology but who are appliance free should continue to have regular urologic follow-up,[2] including residual measurements, roentgenographic studies and measurement of kidney function. The intravenous pyelogram (IVP) and cystourethrogram (CUG) will help identify the presence of calculi, hydronephrosis and reflux as well as other pathology. Kidney function tests (e.g. creatinine or inulin clearance) will evaluate the ability of the kidneys to filter out waste material by measuring the glomerular filtration rate.

When a patient first attains an appliance-free state, measurements of residual urine should be made about once a month for six months. If the amount of residual remains consistently low and no other urinary problems develop, the time between residual checks can be gradually lengthened until they occur annually.

The amount of residual urine that is acceptable will vary with bladder capacity. The goal should be to maintain a residual volume that is less than the *critical residual volume (CRV)*. The critical residual volume is that volume of residual urine below which the bladder is hydrodynamically self-sterilizing. To self-sterilize means that the bladder is capable of effectively washing out any bacterial population; this ability is dependent upon the growth rate (doubling time) of the bacteria, the rate of urine flow and the consistency of the residual volumes. The critical residual urine volume then will depend upon the ability of a person to increase urine production, decrease residual volumes and prolong the doubling time of the bacteria.[5]

In practice, many clinicians strive for residual volumes of no more than 50 to 100 ml. In a patient with consistently sterile urine, slightly larger urine residual volumes are sometimes considered acceptable.

An increase in residual volume may indicate changes in innervation, bladder contractability, and/or the development of sphincter dyssynergia (i.e. the inability of the external sphincter to relax while the bladder wall is contracting).

Cystitis may also result in an increase in residual volumes as the bladder contractions become less efficient.

It should be kept in mind that urinary tract pathology may exist long before the patient exhibits any symptoms. Recognition and early treatment of such problems can prevent more serious disease.

IMPORTANT THINGS TO REMEMBER ABOUT APPLIANCE-FREE STATE

1. The potential for urinary problems remains even after attaining the appliance-free state. Periodic check-ups including residual measurements are important.
2. Be aware of the signs and symptoms of urinary tract infection. Prompt treatment can prevent more serious problems.
3. Avoid bladder overdistention. If sensation of bladder fullness is absent, adhere to bladder-emptying schedules.
4. Maintain a good consistent fluid intake and adjust bladder-emptying schedule to accommodate changes in fluid intake.
5. Avoid alcohol consumption.
6. If using pharmacological management, adhere to medication schedule.

E.N.

REFERENCES

1. Opitz, J.L.: Bladder retraining: An organized program. *Mayo Clin Proc 51:*367–372, 1976.
2. Barkin, M., Dolfin, D., Herschorn, S., Bharatwal, N., and Comisarow, R.: The urologic care of the spinal cord injury patient. *J Urol 129:*335–338, 1983.
3. Newman, E., and Price, M.: Bacteriuria in patients with spinal cord lesions: Its relationship to urinary drainage appliances. *Arch Phys Med Rehabil 58:*427–430, 1977.
4. Brocklehurst, J.C.: Aging of the human bladder. *Geriatrics 27:*154–166, 1972.
5. Hinman, F., and Cox, C.E.: The voiding vesical defense mechanism: The mathematical effect of residual urine, voiding intervals and volume on bacteriuria. *J Urol 96:*491–498, 1966.

Chapter X

SUPRAVESICAL DIVERSION

Supravesical diversion is a surgical procedure sometimes performed when the bladder must be bypassed for some reason. As a rule, urine flows through the ureter into an artificial bladder that has been constructed from a piece of small or large intestine. From here, it drains to the outside through an opening in the abdominal wall. The procedure was first described by Bricker in 1956 and gained popularity with many adaptations in the succeeding years.[1] Nephrostomy and other methods of diversion are less often encountered and will not be discussed.

Supravesical diversion is used infrequently now but may be indicated for children and adults when other modifications of drainage, including cystoplasty and ureteral reimplantations, have failed to prevent urinary tract deterioration or in the event of carcinoma of the bladder.

INDICATIONS FOR USE

The goal or objective of urinary diversion is to preserve renal function by providing adequate urinary drainage when other methods have failed.

The usual indications for urinary diversion in children are: urinary tract deterioration due to congenital or acquired neurogenic bladders, congenital malformations, obstructive anomalies or trauma.[2] Extrophy of the bladder is occasionally effectively treated by closure or ureterosigmoid diversion; however, frequently complications such as stricture of the anastomosis, recurrent pyelonephritis or chloremic acidosis make ileal diversion necessary to prevent renal deterioration.

Repeated urinary tract infection, uncontrollable incontinence and reflux are conditions which may lead to urinary diversion for children with neurogenic bladders due to spinal bifida or spinal cord injury. Reconstructive surgery is often used to prevent renal deterioration when bladder neck obstruction with reflux occurs. However, if these procedures fail, diversion may be performed in an effort to preserve renal function.

In adults, supravesical diversion may be necessitated by complications related to the neurogenic bladder, most commonly vesicoureteral reflux with intractable pyelonephritis, hydronephrosis, or parenchymal atrophy.

149

Carcinoma and trauma with progressive upper tract changes are other conditions that can lead to urinary diversion.

TYPES OF URINARY DIVERSION

Over the years, several types of urinary diversion have been developed and new procedures will undoubtedly be devised.

The ileal diversion procedure as first popularized by Bricker[1] used a small piece of the ileum to produce an artificial bladder or urinary conduit (Fig. X-1). The ileum was chosen because of its adequate blood supply and the peristaltic action which propels the urine through the stoma. A properly constructed ileal conduit will provide good drainage with small residuals and low hydrostatic pressure, provided there is no obstruction to outflow. The ureteroileal anastomosis seldom results in stricture or obstruction at the site of the new ureteral orifice but does not prevent the reflux of potentially infected urine from the ileal conduit into the ureters—a condition that contributes to one of the complications of this method of urinary drainage, namely, pyelonephritis.

The sigmoid conduit was developed to allow for a more easily constructed

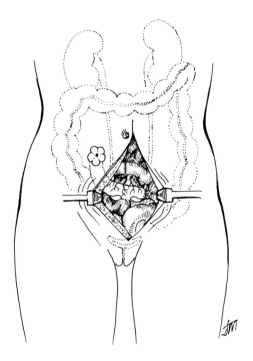

Figure X-1. Surgical procedures for ileal diversion. Ileal conduit constructed from segment of ileum.

anti-reflux ureteral anastomosis.[3,4] This anti-reflux device protects the kidneys from reflux and prevents the passage of infected urine from the conduit to the kidneys.

Other methods of urinary diversion have been used with varying degrees of success, and research continues to present improvements to overcome difficulties associated with current methods.[5,6]

INHERENT DANGERS

Complications of urinary diversion can be divided into two general classifications, early and late, with the early usually occurring within the first thirty days after surgery.[7]

Early complications relate to the surgical procedure itself and include wound infection and wound dehiscence, conditions that are probably related to the lengthy operative procedure and the transection of the bowel. Ureteral leaks or obstruction require early recognition and repair to avoid serious consequences. Intestinal obstruction, intussusception and peritonitis may also occur.

Late complications include peristomal skin problems, stomal stenosis, reflux, hydronephrosis, hyperchloremic acidosis, upper tract infection, pyocystitis, and renal calculi.

Infection

Infection is the most common late complication. The high incidence of bacteriuria in patients with urinary diversion is probably due to two major sources: first, preexisting foci of infection such as chronic pyelonephritis or renal calculi; second, contamination from external sources gaining access through the stoma. Bacteriuria is especially dangerous in those patients whose urinary diversion was not constructed with an anti-reflux ureteral anastomosis. Without this anti-reflux mechanism, bacteria can freely enter the ureter and eventually reach the kidneys.

Danger Areas

The three main danger areas where bacteria can enter the system are the stoma area, the ostomy appliance, and the tubing and urine collecting appliance (leg bag, night bag or jug) (Fig X-2).

Stoma Area: Obstruction to the flow of urine away from the stoma will allow urine to pool and bacteria to multiply (Fig. X-2A). This danger has been reduced somewhat with the use of anti-reflux anastomosis procedures

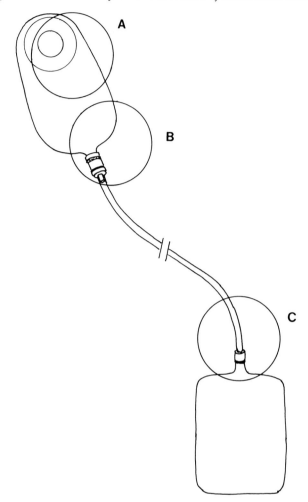

Figure X-2. Danger areas where bacteria can enter the system. A. Stoma area. B. Ostomy appliance. C. Tubing and urine collecting appliance.

in colonic or sigmoid conduits.[3] Tight clothing over the stoma can prevent the conduit from emptying.

Ostomy Appliance: Urine flowing away from the stoma area can also be obstructed by twisting of appliances, plugging of drainage openings or improperly fitted appliances. Using "dirty" appliances will contribute to the high concentration of bacteria in the stoma area (Fig. X-2B).

Tubing and Collecting Appliance: The tubing and collecting appliance (leg bag, night bag or jug) should be washed and disinfected daily to minimize bacterial growth and decrease odor problems (Fig. X-2C) (see Chap. XI, "Disinfection Procedures"). Appliance care is particularly important for patients who are experiencing frequent urinary tract infections. The leg bag and night collecting device must always be kept below the level of the stoma and ostomy pouch to prevent urine from flowing back into the pouch. See Chapter XI for complete instructions on care and positioning of appliances.

Calculi

There is an unusually high incidence of renal calculi in patients with urinary diversions,[8] with reports ranging from 4.7 percent to 30 percent.[9] The incidence varies with the method of urinary diversion and the types of stones formed. Calcium oxalate and struvite calculi form frequently because of increased calcium excretion, large volume of conduit residuals, pre-existing pyelonephritis and the presence of urease-producing micro-organisms.[9] It has been suggested that the construction of the conduit changes the physiologic environment and thereby increases the potential for calculus formation in patients with ileal diversion.[9]

Methods of prevention must be directed to the clinical and physiological conditions leading to stone formation.

Infection can be lessened by proper hygiene and appliance care, but once established it must be vigorously treated, especially if urea-splitting organisms are present. There should be a proper acid-base balance to restore and maintain urine acidity. Conduit revision may be necessary to reduce contact time with intestinal mucosa and large residual volumes which facilitate chloride and bicarbonate exchange.[9]

Uric acid calculi occur more readily in an acid urine. If such calculi are forming, alkalinization may be required to reduce their incidence. See Chapters IV and XVII for more information on bladder and renal calculi.

Stomal Pathology

Stomal complications occur after ileal diversion in approximately 30 percent of all cases.[10,11] The incidence of stomal complications is less frequent with colonic diversion, partly because the lumen of the colon is larger and some degree of constriction can occur without stenosis developing.[4] Other causative factors leading to stomal complications include: improper placement of stoma, non-protruding stoma, inadequate or injurious placement of appliances and failure to maintain an acid urine.

Peristomal Denudement

A flush or non-protruding stoma allows urine to undermine the appliance leading to denudement and a hyperplastic response with thickening of the skin as well as stomal stricture.

Treatment: Change the ostomy appliance more frequently and seek advice from a physician or enterostomal therapist.

Peristomal Dermatitis

Erythematous, denuded, weeping areas around the stoma result from urine "burn," almost always the result of an ill-fitting or improperly applied collecting device. On occasion, the dermatitis may be due to a reaction to adhesive agents.

Treatment: Measure stoma and compare with opening in appliance to insure proper fit. If dermatitis does not improve, help should be obtained from an enterostomal therapist, experienced nurse or physician.

Stomal Bleeding and Encrustation

Stomal bleeding and encrustation is usually the result of alkaline urine and/or unclean collection appliances.

Treatment: Acidify urine with medications and diet. The pH of the urine should be less than 6.5. Clean and change ostomy appliances more frequently. White vinegar can be used to bathe and soak the area. When the appliance has been removed, saturate one or two rayon balls with full-strength white vinegar and apply to stoma and affected skin. Renew saturated rayon balls every five minutes 2 or 3 times. Rinse with plain water and dry well. Replace appliance. One ounce of white vinegar may be instilled into the pouch two to four times a day. Be sure the vinegar comes into contact with all the surface of the pouch. Increase fluid intake unless medically contra-indicated. Use straight drainage with a leg bag, night bag or jug to help minimize urine pooling in the stoma area.

Stoma Stenosis

There have been reports of stricture occurring in from 6–33 percent of all patients with urinary diversions.[11] Stomal stenosis is probably more common in children with ileal diversion, probably because of a greater sensitivity of the skin and the small size of the ileum.[4] Repeated revisions may be necessary until the child is full grown. Other conditions leading to stomal stenosis include an alkaline urine, poor blood supply, excessive skin growth, poor stoma construction, or inappropriate location of stoma on the abdomen.

Treatment: If stenosis is due to inflammation of the bowel segment from alkaline urine, urine acidification may resolve the problem. Often, surgical revision is necessary[12] if renal impairment is to be prevented.

Bladder Complications

The isolated bladder is often left in place when a urinary diversion is performed, usually to reduce an already lengthy operating time. As a rule, the isolated bladder will contract and provide no problems for the patient. Occasionally, however, the bladder will continue to be infected and periodically discharge purulent exudate. If this occurs, a physician should be contacted. Sometimes, the infection will respond to irrigations with sterile saline or antibiotics, but bladder excision is often required. If left untreated, the infection may become severe and in the quadriplegic population could lead to autonomic dysreflexia.

The association of bladder cancer with long-term catheterization has been well recognized, but carcinoma may also develop in the isolated bladder.[13] It should be suspected in patients with repeated bloody purulent urethral discharge. Cystocopy and bladder washing with cytologic examination will aid in its early detection.

Psychological Problems

Urinary diversion produces a change in body structure and body image which can be very frightening to an individual contemplating urinary diversion as well as after surgery.[14] Many questions will need to be addressed. The patient may wonder if the surgery will affect their performance at work or school, as well as their social activity. They will be concerned about sexual inadequacy or undesirability and embarrassment because of spillage. It is important that all health care professionals be aware of these concerns and help the patient adjust to changes in body image by carefully answering questions, providing adequate instruction and giving support.

EFFECT OF DIET AND FLUID INTAKE

Unless medically contraindicated, an adult with a urinary diversion should consume enough liquid to insure an output of approximately 2,000 ml per day. Generally, the best fluids to drink are water and cranberry juice, with an avoidance of those liquids that tend to alkalinize the urine (e.g. orange juice, lemonade, soda pop) (see "Alkaline Ash Diet" in the Appendix). An exception would be those patients who are known to form the uric acid stones which develop more readily in an acid urine. For those people, urine alkalinization is desirable in spite of the other disadvantages. A person who remains free of urinary tract infections and calculi should require no special dietary restrictions to maintain good kidney function.

APPLIANCES

There are many varieties of ostomy appliances. They are available in two general types, either completely disposable or with parts that are reusable. It is not our intention to recommend one type over another but, rather, to suggest the factors to be considered when selecting an ostomy appliance.

All will consist of two general parts: (1) a *face plate, disc* or *mounting ring* that attaches to the body over the stoma and (2) a *pouch* to collect the urine. It is important that the opening in the face plate or disc be the correct size to accommodate the stoma. If it is too small, the disc will cover a portion of the stoma, and if it is too large, the skin around the stoma will be exposed to irritating urine.

Reusable Face Plates

The rubber-type face plates (Fig. X-3) are reusable and come in various sizes and shapes (i.e. round, oval, concave, convex and flat). The choice will depend upon body contour. This kind of face plate has a raised portion around the stoma area which tends to protect the stoma itself from direct pressure from clothing. However, it also allows urine to pool in the recessed area and provides a source of bacteria. Crusty material frequently collects on the edges around the stoma opening, particularly if the urine is alkaline, requiring vigorous cleansing. These face plates are relatively expensive, however, with proper care they can be reused for several months. The face plates should be washed well and disinfected with alcohol before reuse.

Disposable Appliances

Reusable face plates are attached to pouches which are connected to drainage tubing. The pouches are disposable and should be discarded each time the ostomy appliance is replaced (Fig. X-3). The reusable face plate can be attached to the skin by a variety of methods. A double-faced disc may be used. This is a thin paper-like material with adhesive on both sides (Fig. X-3). One side attaches to the face plate and the other to the skin. Some patients use a skin bond which is a glue-like substance that is painted on to the face plate and skin. Another method frequently used is a thin layer of wax-like material which may be cut to the correct size, applied to the face plate and then to skin (e.g. Stomahesive®). The substance has a healing effect when applied over irritated skin. This sort of adhesive generally does not adhere to the skin for as long a period of time as the other kinds, necessitating more frequent appliance changes. Patients may use more than one type of adhesive together.

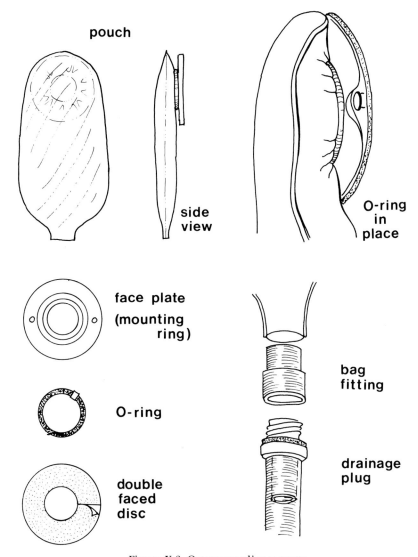

pouch

side view

O-ring in place

face plate (mounting ring)

O-ring

double faced disc

bag fitting

drainage plug

Figure X-3. Ostomy appliance parts.

In addition to the type of appliance with a reusable face plate, there are several completely disposable appliances available. These are a good alternative when a patient has recurring urinary tract infections. Most consist of a pouch with an adhesive disc attached. They are easy to apply and eliminate the necessity of cleansing and disinfecting parts, as the entire bag is discarded (Fig. X-4). Most are flat and the stoma protrudes into the bag, so care must be taken not to injure the stoma with clothing. Some patients apply paper tape around the edge of the mounting ring for additional security. Be sure to check for skin irritation from the tape.

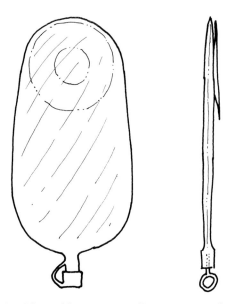

Figure X-4. Disposable ostomy appliance. Front and side view.

Leg Bag Tubing and Night Drainage Appliances

Most ostomy pouches come with an emptying spout, which may be closed and opened to collect and drain the urine. This drainage spout may also be attached to a piece of tubing and a leg bag or night bag (Figs. X-3 & X-5). It is recommended that persons with long-term urinary problems, particularly those with decreased mobility and frequent urinary tract infections, use the additional tubing and bag for urine collection. Continuous drainage will provide a more rapid flow of urine away from the stoma, reducing the chance of urine pooling around the stoma, the ostomy pouch overfilling, and back pressure developing into the conduit.

The tubing and leg bag or night bag should always be kept below the level of the stoma and ostomy pouch. The tubing, leg bag and night drainage system should be disinfected daily (see Chapter XI, "Disinfection Procedure").

CARE PROCEDURES

The ostomy appliance (pouch and face plate) should be removed and replaced at least every four to five days. If using a reusable face plate, all

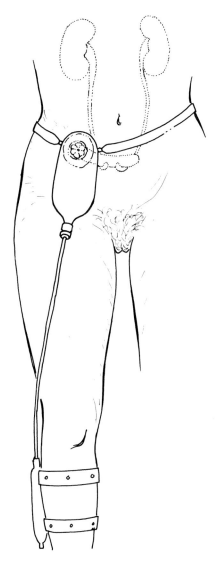

Figure X-5. Ostomy pouch connected to tubing and leg bag for continuous drainage.

adhesive should be removed and it should be cleaned and disinfected with 70 percent alcohol before reuse. Be sure all encrustations are removed from the center opening in the face plate. If they cannot be removed, the face plate should be discarded to prevent stomal injury and infection. The pouch should be discarded. Any adaptors, plugs, etc., used to attach the pouch to the tubing should be washed free from all encrustation and disinfected with 70 percent alcohol (see Chap. XI, "Alcohol Disinfection").

If disposable pouches with disposable mounting rings are being used, they should be discarded when removed and new ones used. The tubing, leg bag and night drainage bag or jug should be disinfected daily (see Chap. XI, "Disinfection Procedure"). Tubing, leg bags, and night bags or jugs should be replaced frequently—ideally, once a week but at least once a month.

Frequent checking of equipment to insure unobstructed urine flow from the conduit to urine collecting bag or jug will help eliminate potential problems.

Odor often becomes a problem for patients with urinary diversion. Since odor is primarily due to bacterial action, it can sometimes be lessened by flushing the ostomy bag once or twice a day with a dilute povidone-iodine solution (1 part povidone-iodine solution to 5 parts boiled water), in addition to meticulous care of the collecting apparatus. If the patient is allergic to povidone-iodine, white vinegar may be used.

Directions for Ostomy Bag Flush

1. Detach the tubing from the ostomy appliance and squirt or pour a small amount of diluted povidone-iodine or white vinegar into the open end of the ostomy appliance.
2. Swish this solution around inside the bag, allowing it to flow around the stoma area.
3. Re-attach the tubing and allow the solution to flow out of the ostomy bag as new urine is formed.

This procedure can easily be accomplished in the morning and evening when changing drainage systems from night equipment (night bag or jug) to day equipment (leg bag) and vice versa.

Povidone-iodine is virtually non-toxic and non-sensitizing, although an occasional person will be allergic to the iodine component. It is a bacterial suppressant which helps to minimize the number of bacteria surrounding the stoma area. If skin irritation should result, discontinue use and consult a physician or enterostomal therapist. Vinegar also has some anti-bacterial properties and is inexpensive.

Anti-Twist Device

Patients with urinary diversions, especially quadriplegics with limited hand function, often have difficulty keeping their ostomy appliance from twisting and preventing the flow of urine through the tubing into the collecting bag. The resultant filling of the ostomy bag will permit urine to pool around the stoma and eventually produce back pressure, causing distention of the urinary conduit. Reflux of contaminated urine into the conduit, ureter and kidneys can lead to pyelonephritis. The weight and pressure from the overfilled pouch may also pull the appliance away from the skin, leading to wet clothing or bedding and causing embarrassment to the patient.

There are some ostomy pouches available with "built-in" anti-twist devices. With others, an anti-twist device can be added by attaching a piece of lightweight cardboard or adhesive one-eighth-inch foam to the pouch. The reinforcement should be cut in the shape of the lower end of the bag and attached to the bag by adhesive or tape. This adds enough firmness to the pouch to resist twisting (Fig X-6).

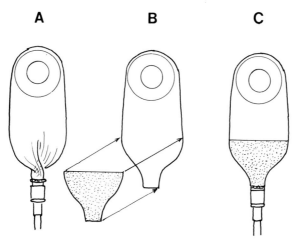

Figure X-6. Anti-twist device for ostomy pouch. See text for instructions.

Body Support Garments

If a patient is wearing an abdominal binder or corset, care must be taken to prevent obstruction of urine flow. A hole can be cut in the corset to accommodate the ostomy appliance (Fig. X-7) or strips of foam (approx. 1/2" × 1/2" × 4") can be placed on each side of the stoma to remove pressure from the stoma (Fig. X-7). Sometimes a support garment with an appropriate opening for the appliance actually aids in keeping the appliance intact and improves length of wearing time.

Observation

Much information can be gained about the function and fit of an ostomy appliance by careful observation. A good time to examine the stoma area is when the ostomy pouch has been removed to change appliances or to obtain

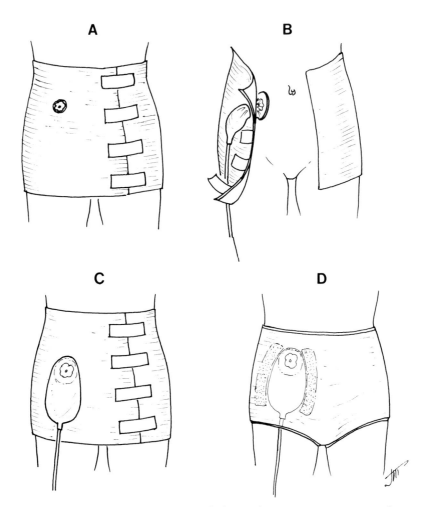

Figure X-7. Body support garments. A. A hole cut in garment to accommodate ostomy appliance. B. Ostomy appliance being placed through the opening in garment. C. Appliance in place. D. Foam strips placed along sides of appliance to reduce pressure on the stoma from clothing.

a urine specimen for culture. After the pouch has been removed, gently clean the area around the stoma, look for areas of abrasion and erythema. Measure the stoma and check the size of the ring opening. Is it too small, overlapping the stoma, or too large, allowing urine to bathe the skin around the stoma? Does the stoma and adjacent skin bleed on the slightest contact? Are there encrustations on and/or around the stoma? Select a correct size face plate and treat any stomal pathology.

Observe the urine flow and the length of time between flows of urine. This will give you a good idea of the peristaltic action of the loop. Conduit residual can be measured by passing a sterile catheter into the conduit immediately after a urine flow, aspirating the urine remaining in the conduit. Conduit residual should be measured routinely whenever it is catheterized to obtain a specimen for urine culture (see Chapter XII, "Culture Procedures"). Large residuals may indicate problems with stomal strictures or a stretched and sagging conduit.

Is the stoma so tight that it is difficult to pass a catheter? If so, it may indicate the need for medical/surgical intervention. Report this to the physician.

ENTEROSTOMAL THERAPISTS

Enterostomal therapists are experienced registered nurses who have completed a postgraduate nursing specialty program. They are knowledgeable and trained in the preoperative and postoperative management of patients with ostomies and provide a valuable resource for patients and health care professionals. For information regarding enterostomal therapists in your area, contact:

> International Association of Enterostomal Therapy
> 505 North Tustin Avenue, Suite 219
> Santa Ana, California 92705
> (714) 541-5227

IMPORTANT THINGS TO REMEMBER ABOUT
SUPRAVESICAL DIVERSION URINARY DRAINAGE

1. Always wash hands vigorously before and after drainage appliance care.
2. Ostomy pouch should be changed about every five days. Remove appliance carefully to avoid skin abrasion. Sometimes, it is necessary to use adhesive remover.
3. Before reapplying an ostomy pouch, wash area well and remove with a razor or scissors any hair growing in area where the pouch is to be attached.
4. Check stoma area for skin irritations or lesions. If noted, consult physician or enterostomal therapist.
5. If a reusable mounting ring is used, be sure it has been thoroughly cleansed.
6. Attach appliance to skin using appropriate procedure for each patient.
7. Use a continuous drainage system (i.e. tubing and a leg bag or night bag or jug) to allow urine to drain away from ostomy pouch. An

overfilled ostomy pouch will cause back pressure on the stoma and the loop and can pull the pouch loose from the skin. It may also push contaminated urine back into the loop and up to the kidneys.

8. If continuous drainage is not used, empty pouch frequently to avoid overfilling and back pressure on stoma.

9. Tubing, leg bag and night drainage system should be rinsed, washed with detergent, rinsed and disinfected daily (see Chap. XI, "Disinfection Procedure").

10. Care must be taken to prevent the ostomy pouch from twisting, thereby preventing outflow of urine (see anti-twist device).

11. Position tubing, leg bag and/or night bag or jug below level of ostomy pouch. Do not allow urine to flow back toward stoma area. Be sure tubing is correct length and that leg bag when used is in proper position.

12. Flushing ostomy pouch daily with povidone-iodine solution will help reduce bacterial growth and odor. If the patient is allergic to povidone-iodine solution, white vinegar may be used, but we have found this to be less effective.

13. Encourage good consistent fluid intake.

E.N.

REFERENCES

1. Bricker, E.M.: Substitution for urinary bladder by use of isolated ileal segments. *Surg Clin North Amer 36*:1117–1130, 1956.
2. Logan C.W., Scott, R. Jr., and Laskowski, T.Z.: Ileal loop diversion: Evaluation of late results in pediatric urology. *J Urol 94*:544–548, 1965.
3. Scardino, P.T., Bagley, D.H., Javadpour, N., and Ketcham, A.: Sigmoid conduit urinary diversion. *Urol 6*:167–170, 1975.
4. Kelalis, P.P.: Urinary diversion in children by the sigmoid conduit: Its advantages and limitations. *J Urol 112*:666–673, 1974.
5. Skinner, D.G.: In search of the ideal method of urinary diversion (guest editorial). *J Urol 128*:476, 1982
6. Beckley, S., Wajsman, Z., Pontes, J.E., and Murphy, G.: Transverse colon conduit: a method of urinary diversion after pelvic radiation. *J Urol 128*:464–468, 1982
7. Remigailo, R.V., Lewis, E.L., Woodard, J.R., and Walton, K.N.: Ileal conduit urinary diversion. Ten-year review. *Urol 7*:343–344, 1976
8. Reisner, G.S., Wilansky, D.L., and Schneiderman, C.: Uric acid lithiasis in the ileostomy patient. *Brit J Urol 45*:340–343, 1973
9. Dretler, S.P.: The pathogenesis of urinary tract calculi occurring after ileal conduit diversion: I. Clinical Study. II. Conduit Study. III. Prevention. *J Urol 109*:204–209, 1973
10. Markland, C., and Flochs, R.H.: The ileal conduit stoma. *J Urol 95*:344–349, 1966
11. Richardson, J.R., Linton, P.C., and Leadbetter, G.W. Jr.: A new concept in the treatment of stomal stenosis. *J Urol 108*:159–161, 1972

12. Derrick, W.A., and Hodges, C.V.: Ileal conduit stasis: Recognition, treatment and prevention. *J Urol 107*:747:750, 1972
13. Rege, P.R., and Evans, A.T.: Carcinoma in isolated bladder after ileoconduit diversion. *Urol 5*:652–653, 1975.
14. Prudden, J.F.: Psychological problems following ileostomy and colostomy. *Cancer 24*:236–238, 1971

Chapter XI

INFECTION—INCIDENCE, PREVENTION AND CONTROL

BACTERIURIA, INCIDENCE AND ORGANISM ISOLATION PATTERNS

U rinary tract infections occur in humans in gradually increasing frequency as age increases. In females, this change is not notable until the sexually active years are reached and pregnancies occur.[1] Bacteriuria has been reported to range from 1.1 percent in school-age girls to 2.3 percent in ages fifteen to thirty-nine years and 10 percent in women at sixty years and older.[2]

Males, on the other hand, appear to maintain a lower infection rate until about age sixty to seventy, when prostatic pathology and urethral strictures lead to an increase in incidence from 0.03 percent to 0.5 percent.[2] In hospitalized males over the age of seventy, incidences as high as 15 percent have been reported.[2]

There is a marked increase in bacteriuria in diabetic women (18%) and diabetic men (5%), as well as a dramatic increase in the aged population with chronic or debilitating diseases, in the disabled and in the chronically ill.[2, 3]

Data collected during renal function evaluations of our population of patients with spinal cord injuries during the period from 1976–1981 reveal a high percentage of patients demonstrating bacteriuria. Sixty-four percent of the total population had bacteriuria, with a range of 21 percent for patients who were appliance free to 97 percent of those using suprapubic catheters (Table XI-I).

The organism isolation pattern obtained for this population of patients differs from that of the general population[3–5] and reflects what could be expected from persons with neurogenic bladders or long-term urinary problems of whatever etiology (Table XI-II).

People with long-term urinary problems will often have multiple species of organisms in their urine compounding the problem of treatment, since each different species of organisms present may have a different sensitivity pattern. It will be noted from the study of Table XI-I that only those patients who were appliance-free had but one species of organism present.

There is some difference of opinion as to what represents a significant colony count as discussed in Chapter XII. It is our belief that colony counts of less than 100,000 colonies per/ml often are significant. In our population

TABLE XI-I

INCIDENCE AND CONCENTRATION OF ORGANISMS OCCURRING IN URINE CULTURES FROM
PATIENTS WITH SPINAL CORD LESIONS (1976-1980)*

Culture Results		Total	MODE OF DRAINAGE						
			Ind. Cath.	Supra. Cath.	Ileal Diver.	Ext. Cath.	Appl. Free	Inter** Cath.	OTHER
Number of Patients		909	259	78	249	139	138	40	6
Positive Cultures	No.	579	232	76	139	76	29	22	6
	%	63.7	89.6	97.4	55.8	54.7	21.0	55.0	100.0
Positive with Multiple Species	%	56.6	73.7	82.9	59.0	32.9	0	31.8	83.3
Species per Postive Culture									
1 Species	%	43.4	26.3	17.1	57.6	67.1	100.0	68.2	16.7
2 Species	%	24.7	30.2	27.6	20.9	22.4	0	31.8	16.7
3 Species	%	16.0	21.1	26.3	12.9	5.3	0	0	50.0
4+ Species	%	15.8	22.4	28.9	8.6	5.3	0	0	16.7
Mean Number per Positive Culture		2.2	2.6	2.9	1.7	1.5	1	1.3	2.8
Range		1-7	1-7	1-7	1-5	1-4	1	1-2	1-5
Concentration (Colonies per ml)									
100,000 & Greater	%	51.4	53.0	50.0	33.5	73.5	55.2	65.5	70.6
10,000-99,000	%	27.0	27.4	28.4	34.3	15.9	3.4	13.8	23.5
1,000-9,000	%	15.4	15.2	15.3	23.6	6.2	17.2	10.3	5.9
1,000	%	6.2	4.3	6.3	8.7	4.4	24.1	10.3	0

*Patients Seen at Renal Function Follow-up Univ. of Mn. Hospitals
**1979–1980
Key: Ind. Cath. = Indwelling Catheter, Supra. Cath. = Suprapubic Catheter, Ileal Diver. = Ileal Diversion, Appl. Free = Appliance Free, Inter. Cath. = Intermittent Catheters

of patients, only one-half of the pathogenic organisms occurring in cultures were present in concentration of 100,000 col/ml or greater (Table XI-I). Our patients frequently were symptomatic with colony counts of less than 100,000 col/ml. Table XI-II demonstrates the differences in organism isolation patterns for persons from different populations and different localities. It is of interest to note the lower percentage of *E. coli* and higher percentage of *Pseudomonas* and alpha hemolytic streptococci occurring in the spinal cord injury group compared to the other groups. This is in keeping with the knowledge that persons with neurogenic bladders or with histories of urinary tract instrumentation and long-term drainage problems are subject to infections with species of bacteria which do not ordinarily cause urinary tract infections in normal, healthy individuals.

Relationship of Method of Urinary Drainage

Table XI-III further differentiates the organism isolation pattern with the method of urinary drainage in use by these patients.

TABLE XI-II
PERCENT OF COMPARISONS OF CULTURE RESULTS
FROM DIFFERENT POPULATIONS OF PATIENTS
Organisms occurring in Cultures in Concentrations of 100,000 col/ml or Greater

Organism	Newman[1] SCI 1976–80	Needham[2] Hospital Population	Mulholland[3] Hospital Population	Mulholland[3] Community Acquired	Franzblau[4] Community Acquired
Escherichia coli	20.8	35.2	26	35	72
Proteus mirabilis	6.9	9.7			
Proteus sp.			17	16	14
(not mirabilis)	8.4	2.7			
Alpha streptococci enterococcus	15.3	9.7	8	10	
Klebsiella	9.4	18.7	15	13	10*
Pseudomonas aeruginosa	16.6	6.9	12	5	4
Staphlococcus (coag +)	2.8	2.3			
Staphlococcus (coag −)	2.2	3.4			
Providencia	3.2	1.7			
Enterobacter	2.3	3.0	7	7	
Serratia	3.1	0.3	7	3	
Other	9.0	6.4	8	11	
TOTAL NUMBER OF ORGANISMS	1259	1,053	525	695	

*Klebsiella-Enterobacter Group
1. Newman – Spinal Cord Lesion (SCL) Patients, U. of Minnesota Hospitals 1976–1980.
2. Needham – General Hospital Population U. of Minnesota. 1962–1968 *J. Urol 104*:831–832, 1970.
3. Mulholland, U. of Pennsylvania. *J. Urol 110*:245–248, 1973.
4. Franzblau, New Mexico. *Urology* 6:30–33, 1975.

Indwelling and Suprapubic Catheters

In patients with indwelling urethral or suprapubic catheters, the organism occurring most frequently is *Pseudomonas* (Table XI-III). You will recall that *Pseudomonas* is not usually found in the intestinal tract of humans, and their presence in a urine culture strongly suggests contamination from external sources. Improper handling of drainage appliance, improper cleansing of drainage equipment, and uncleanliness of self all contributed to bacteriuria from exogenous sources.

Let's review briefly the material in Chapters V and VI. There are three major sources of bacteriuria in patients with indwelling urethral and suprapubic catheters. First, the point of entry of the catheter, the catheterization process itself and the perineal or stoma area. Second, the catheter-tubing union, which must be vigorously wiped with alcohol or povidone-iodine

TABLE XI-III
PERCENT OF INCIDENTS OF ORGANISMS OCCURRING IN ANY CONCENTRATION
IN URINE CULTURES FROM PATIENTS WITH SPINAL CORD LESIONS
(JANUARY 1, 1976–DECEMBER 31, 1980)*

| | | MODE OF DRAINAGE | | | | | |
Organism	Total	Ind. Cath.	Supra. Cath.	Ileal Diver.	Ext. Cath.	Appl. Free	Inter.** Cath.
Alpha streptococci enterococcus	13.9	16.4	14.9	6.2	11.9	23.3	3.4
Streptococcus sp.	3.1	3.0	6.4	2.0	0.8	0	6.8
Staphylococcus (coag. +)	3.3	2.8	9.5	0.8	1.7	0	3.4
Staphylococcus (coag. −)	4.1	4.2	4.1	1.2	1.7	6.7	24.1
Escherichia coli	18.3	19.4	6.3	17.8	30.5	36.7	27.6
Enterobacter	2.4	1.8	3.2	0.8	5.9	3.3	6.9
Klebsiella	8.4	10.4	7.2	7.4	5.1	0	17.2
Citrobacter	4.2	3.5	3.6	5.8	1.7	6.7	0
Providence	2.5	2.0	1.8	4.5	0.8	0	3.4
Serratia	2.8	2.5	4.1	1.2	5.1	0	0
Pseudomonas aeruginosa	17.6	17.4	20.3	19.0	16.9	3.3	3.4
Pseudomonas sp.	0.7	0.4	0.5	0	2.5	3.3	3.4
Proteus mirabilis	7.4	3.8	6.3	18.2	5.1	6.7	0
Proteus vulgaris	1.0	0.8	0.5	2.9	1.7	0	0
Proteus morganii	2.7	2.2	4.1	2.9	2.5	0	0
Providencia rettgeri	3.0	3.0	2.7	4.5	2.5	0	0
Candida	1.9	4.5	0.9	0.4	0.8	3.3	0
Other	2.5	1.7	4.1	4.1	2.5	6.7	0
TOTAL Number of Organisms	1,259	598	222	242	118	30	29

*Patients Seen at Time of Annual Renal Function Follow-up University of Minnesota Hospitals.
**1979 and 1980 only.

Key: Ind. Cath. = Indwelling Catheter, Supra. Cath. = Suprapubic Catheter, Ileal Diver. = Ileal Diversion, Appl. Free = Applicance Free, Inter. Cath. = Intermittent Catheters

before separation. It was because of the danger of contamination in that area that the closed urinary drainage system was developed. The third danger area is the tubing and urine collecting appliance. Care must be taken to always keep the equipment below the level of the bladder to permit prompt drainage of urine from the bladder and to prevent backflow of urine from the appliance through the catheter into the bladder. The drainage appliance should be adequately disinfected daily to minimize bacterial contamination.

Ileal Diversion

The high incidence of bacteriuria in patients with urinary diversion is reason for concern, since most patients with diversion have some degree of reflux from the urinary conduit to the kidneys. One of the sources of infection is the backflow of urine from the collecting appliance into the conduit and then up the ureters to the kidneys. Consequently, it is imperative that the urine drain away from the stoma area. Twisting of the ostomy appliance and too tight clothing must be avoided, since the high incidence of *Pseudomonas* suggests contamination from external sources (Table XI-III). Ostomy pouches should be changed frequently and appliances disinfected daily. The frequent finding of *Proteus mirabilis* is further reason for concern, since *P. mirabilis* is a urea splitter and will tend to alkalinize the urine, which may encourage bacterial growth, irritate the skin in the stoma area and could lead to calculus formation.

External Catheters

Since the use of external catheters is a non-invasive method of urinary tract drainage, it could be anticipated that the incidence of bacteriuria would be low; yet, our studies show that 55 percent had bacteriuria. One-third of these cultures contained more than one species of organism, with a high incidence of *Pseudomonas* (17%) (Table XI-III), again indicating contamination of the drainage system from exogenous sources. The higher incidence of *E. coli* (31%), an organism of endogenous source, would suggest uncleanliness of self with a transfer of *E. coli* from the intestinal tract to the urinary tract. Good perineal care, consistent handwashing, and maintenance of dryness in the perineal area will help to eliminate this source. The external catheter should be changed daily and urine collecting appliances disinfected daily. Care must be taken to prevent urine from pooling in the external catheter because of improper placement of appliance, twisting or kinking of the appliance, or a full drainage bag.

Intermittent Catheterization

A 55 percent incidence of bacteriuria in our spinal cord injured population using intermittent catheterization is much higher than expected. Although all of these patients were instructed and maintained on a sterile and frequent catheterization regimen while in the hospital, it is probable that deviation from sterile procedures, plus overdistention as the result of too infrequent catheterizing, leads to this high incidence of bacteriuria. Other investigations have reported similar high percentages.[6,7] The organisms occurring most frequently were *E. coli,* coagulase-negative *Staphylococcus* and *Klebsiella,* all organisms that are normal to the intestinal tract or skin, suggesting the sources of contamination (Table XI-III).

Appliance Free

Surprisingly, 21 percent of our appliance-free patients exhibited positive urine cultures, although only one species of bacteria was present in each of their cultures. There are several possible explanations for the number of infections. First, since these patients all had neurogenic bladders and had experienced urinary drainage problems, it is possible that the bladder's natural defense mechanism was not functioning adequately, allowing bacteria to become established in the bladder. Second, to avoid incontinence or the need to urinate frequently, fluid intake may have been restricted and bacteria washout made ineffective. Third, chronic infections existing prior to attaining the appliance-free state may perpetuate infection.

NOSOCOMIAL INFECTIONS

Nosocomial infection is a term used in relation to infection acquired within a hospital. In a broader sense, it applies to extended health care facilities and nursing homes. There are thousands of nosocomial infections reported each year, at an estimated annual cost of over two billion dollars. Over one-half of these infections involve the urinary tract.[8] Nosocomial infections are often more difficult and expensive to treat because they occur in an environment where pathogenic antibiotic-resistant organisms are prevalent.

Sources

Commercially Prepared Products

Catheter kits with contaminated disinfectant packets, catheter irrigation kits, IV sets and other commercially prepared materials have been implicated in episodes of hospital infections. An alert staff and infection control personnel will often be able to identify sources through epidemiologic studies. Infection from this type of source are often due to organisms such as *Enterobacter* and *Pseudomonas.*[9, 10]

Contaminated Equipment

Improperly sterilized, stored and/or handled equipment can contribute to infection (e.g. nebulizers and urinals). Urinals interchanged between patients have been shown to contribute to urinary tract infections.[11]

Airborne

Aerosolization from improper handling of contaminated material (e.g. urine and wound drainage) will spread disease. Infections from these sources are often due to highly resistant Gram-negative rods such as *E. coli, Proteus* and *Pseudomonas. Skin scales* rubbed off on bedding, clothing, etc., can easily become airborne, carrying microorganisms from one area to another.

Contact

Contact can be direct from one patient to another or indirect from a patient to an object, then to another patient or to an intermediary person and then to the patient. Hands usually play an active role in all of these types of contact.

Hands

Since handwashing is a relatively inexpensive, simple effective control of the spread of infection, one wonders why it is not more frequently used. Studies have demonstrated that in two types of medical intensive care units the number of health care professionals who washed their hands after direct contact with the patients ranged from 28–41 percent.[12]

Handwashing facilities, preferably with knee or foot controls, should be available in all areas where there will be patient contact. Good antiseptic soaps or detergents should be conveniently located. Hands should be washed vigorously front, back and between the fingers. Brush scrubbing is usually reserved for surgical scrubbing. Rinse hands well and dry on paper towels. Hand-operated faucets should be turned off holding paper towels. WASH YOUR HANDS AFTER EVERY PATIENT CONTACT.

Other Objects

There are many other things to consider as contact sources of infection, such as clothing, bedding, soap dishes, faucets, plants and curtains, as well as invasive devices such as IV's and catheters. The privacy curtains used around patient beds often become contaminated when they are open and closed by contaminated hands. Curtains, bedding and clothing may become contaminated from spilled urine, drainage from infected wounds or fecal material. Careless handling of these items will then transfer microorganisms to the surrounding environment. Plants and vases of flowers can be a reservoir for microorganisms such as *Pseudomonas cepacia, Pseudomonas pseudomallei, Serratia* and *Erwina,* as all are species known to inhabit soil or stagnant water. Although these are organisms that are usually not pathogenic to the normal population, they can cause infection in patients with reduced resistance. All have been found in urine cultures. Care must be taken to wash hands after testing the soil of plants for dryness or vases to determine water levels.

It is recommended that, when possible, two persons with indwelling catheters not be placed in the same room. Makie and co-workers[13] have demonstrated that microorganisms present in the urine of one patient with an indwelling catheter will be present in the urine of a roommate with an indwelling catheter within seventy-two hours.

To control the incidence of nosocomial infections, it is essential that health care facilities develop and enforce good infection control measures and good quality control in sterilizing and supply units.

COMMUNITY-ACQUIRED INFECTIONS

Most of the preceding information will also apply directly to the prevention of infection in community settings (e.g. private homes). Some additional precautions also apply whether you live in the home to provide care or visit periodically (e.g. public health nurse).

Washing hands before or after patient contact is just as essential. Although the bacteria normally present in a household are less apt to be as pathogenic or antibiotic resistant as those in a hospital, they may still pose a threat to the susceptible patient. Health care professionals coming into the home may carry pathogenic organisms from a previous patient contact.

Handwashing in patients' homes may not always be as convenient as in a hospital. It is a good idea to bring along a supply of paper towels and detergent.

Care must be taken when transporting supplies and equipment to prevent contamination through broken seals, punctured packages, etc.

Clean up well before leaving the home. Place all contaminated items in a plastic bag (bring one with you) for proper disposal. *Wash hands before leaving.*

DISINFECTION, STERILIZATION AND APPLIANCE CARE

To correctly use various chemical and physical agents available today, an understanding of the terminology is helpful.

Definition of Terms

Disinfectant: An antimicrobial agent that frees from infection by either killing the microorganism or preventing it from growing. It may or may not be effective against spores. The term *disinfectant* is usually reserved for those agents that are effective against inanimate objects. Action of some may be influenced by time, concentration, temperature and pH.

Antiseptic: An antimicrobial agent which frees from infection either by killing the microorganism or preventing its growth. It may or may not affect spores. The term *antiseptic* is usually reserved for those agents that are used upon the skin.

Antibiotic: An antimicrobial agent which frees from infection either by killing the microorganism or preventing its growth. These are agents that are usually administered systemically, but some are more appropriately applied to the skin or mucous membranes.

Disinfectants, antiseptics and antibiotics may be selective in their action, being effective against some microorganisms and not others.

Sterilize: Any process, physical or chemical, which will destroy all forms of life, applied especially to microorganisms, including bacterial cells and spores, mold and spores and viruses.

Sanitizer: An agent that reduces microbial contamination. The term does not imply complete disinfection or sterilization. They are commonly used in control of bacterial contamination of floors, furniture, in restaurants and in food processing plants.

Bacteriostatic: Arrests bacterial growth. Bacteria are not killed and growth may resume when bacteriostatic agent is removed.

Bacteriocidal: Kills bacterial cells.

Sporicide: Kills bacterial spores.

Basic Considerations

There are several points to be taken into consideration when planning a disinfection or sterilization procedure.

1. Microorganisms can be irreversibly killed or reversibly inhibited.
2. Various microbial groups differ in their response to sterilizing or inhibiting agents (e.g. spores, young cells, resting cells).

3. Disinfection and sterilization is a function of time. All microorganisms do not die at the same time.
4. Consider the nature and function of the material to be treated.

Physical Agents

Heat

Heat may be used in many different ways to sterilize objects. It is rapid and relatively inexpensive. Two factors must be considered. They are *time* and *temperature*, and they will vary with method. The *thermal death point* is the temperature at which all the microorganisms in a standardized pure culture are killed in a specified time, and the *thermal death time* is the time required to kill all the organisms at a given temperature.

Heat may be either *moist* or *dry*. With high dry heat, components within the microbial cell are oxidized. With lower heat, the oxidation process is very slow. When moist heat is used, the cellular proteins within the bacterial cell are coagulated and the enzymatic function of the protein destroyed. Moist heat will sterilize more quickly and at lower temperatures. In general, moist heat is less damaging to objects being sterilized.

Moist Heat

Hot water applied with force or agitation will *sanitize* an object. The water should be at least 60° C, 140° F, and the presence of detergents will improve the cleansing action by lowering the surface tension. This is not a *disinfection* or *sterilization* process.

Boiling (100° C, 212° F) for thirty minutes will kill vegetative cells, but not spores or viruses, provided the objects are clean. Any residue such as blood or mucus left on objects may coagulate in the heat and protect the bacteria from the heat. Washing items well with detergent and adding detergent to the boiling water will help eliminate this problem. It should be kept in mind that this method will not kill spores and viruses. If complete sterilization is required, some other method should be used.

Steam under pressure or *autoclaving* is a process where steam pressure is increased within a chamber to raise the temperature. A vacuum chamber (autoclave) is used. Steam at 100° C, 212° F flows into the chamber while air is flushed out through an outlet valve. When all the air has been replaced with steam, the valve is closed and steam continues to flow in to increase the pressure until the desired temperature is reached. The temperature and time required is critical and is based on the thermal death time or thermal death point of the microorganism to be eliminated. For example, to kill specific heat-resistant spores, a steam pressure of fifteen pounds per square inch for twelve to fifteen minutes is required, while only three to five minutes are required at thirty pounds pressure.[14] The pressure is maintained for the desired time, the steam is then turned off and the chamber allowed to cool. The items sterilized will require a drying time before use. The chamber must be loaded in the correct manner to allow even penetration of steam. If using this procedure, be sure to follow manufacturer's guidelines carefully. Test organisms are available to check the efficiency of the process.

Dry Heat

Hot air treatment or baking requires a long period of time at a high temperature (e.g. 165° C, 329° F for two hours).[14] Heat penetrates slowly and does not penetrate all objects at the same time. A well-regulated chamber is required which must be packed loosely to allow even circulation of heat. Many objects cannot stand this high a temperature for the prolonged time required, but the method is sometimes used for glassware and metal objects.

Incineration can be used to sterilize and dispose of dispensable contaminated objects. When incineration is used, care must be taken to be sure the chamber is heated sufficiently and that all items are completely burned. Closely packed or moist items frequently require a longer time in the burning chamber.

Other Methods of sterilization have been developed for specific conditions and materials such as ultraviolet, filtration, and sonic disruption. Since these methods are not usually used in relation to urinary tract care, they will not be discussed here.

Chemical Agents

As already discussed, the action of a chemical agent will be affected by the nature of the microorganism, the concentration of the chemical and of the microorganism, the time exposed, the presence of extraneous material and possibly by the pH of the solution.

The chemical nature of the disinfectant will determine its mode of action against the microorganism. The modes of action include: (1) coagulation of the cell protein, (2) denaturing of cellular proteins, (3) oxidation of protein enzymes, and (4) lysing of cells.

Alcohol

Several of the alcohols are bactericidal; however, *ethyl* and *isopropyl* or *propyl* alcohols are most commonly used. (*Methyl* alcohol is *not* effective.) They act against vegetative cells by coagulating or denaturing the protein.

Since water is required for their effectiveness, a 70 percent solution is recommended. Alcohols have the advantage of being rapid in their action against cells. They are relatively inexpensive and evaporate to leave no residue. The fact that they leave no residue may also be a disadvantage. They evaporate rapidly from a surface and, with no residual activity, limit the exposure time. When used as a solution (e.g. in a container), the alcohol will evaporate and leave a higher concentration of water, decreasing the bacteriocidal effect; so alcohol should always be kept in closed containers. For disinfecting urinary appliances, a ten-minute soak of the previously cleansed item in a closed container is recommended to allow sufficient time for the alcohol to penetrate to all surfaces.

Phenols

Phenols are coal tar derivatives and have been used as a disinfectant in various forms and concentrations for years. In high concentrations, phenols act by penetrating and disrupting the cell wall and coagulating cell protein. In lower concentrations the death of the bacterial cell results from inactivation of essential enzyme systems.[15] There are a variety of phenolic disinfectants available, each of which may contain different concentrations of phenol. Read the labels carefully to determine the dilutions to use for *disinfection.* Phenols are generally not effective against spores, although, with increased temperature to 100°C (boiling), some sporicidal activity has been noted. They have the advantage of being effective in a comparatively short time (30-minute contact is recommended for urinary appliances such as leg bags and tubing). They are compatible with soaps and detergents and are not inactivated by organic matter. They have some residual activity if allowed to dry on a surface. Their disadvantage is their corrosive action against metals, their strong odor and the skin irritations they can produce. Some examples are Lysol® and Osyl®.

Surface Active Agents

Surface active agents include the quaternary ammonium compounds, soaps and detergents. They act by lowering the tension between molecules upon a surface. *Quaternary ammonium compounds* are effective against many vegetative bacterial cells but are generally not effective against spores. They act against microbes by disrupting the molecular barriers that hold the cells and the surrounding media apart and expose the interior of the cell to the external environment.

Quaternary ammonium compounds have the advantage of being non-toxic and odorless. They have the disadvantage of being inactivated by soaps and detergents. They are also inhibited by organic matter, as they have a strong affinity for proteins, both plant and animal. Even traces of contamination with organic matter will inactivate a solution. This is particularly important when using a quaternary ammonium compound to disinfect urinary drainage appliances. They must be washed free of organic matter and rinsed free of detergents or soap before disinfection. Since these compounds are also attracted to plant proteins, they should not be used with cotton balls or cotton gauze squares because they will become inactivated by the plant proteins.[14]

Some solutions, particularly if they become contaminated with organic matter, soaps or detergents, will actually support bacterial growth.[14] For this reason, solutions should be made up fresh and discarded after use. An example of a quaternary ammonium compound is Zephiran®.

Soaps and detergents serve as cleaning agents, as they increase the wetability of a surface by lowering surface tension. They enable oils and waters to mix together, allowing debris to be washed off. Soaps have no chemical action upon most normal skin microorganisms. Detergents have a higher degree of surface activity than soaps and some may have a bactericidal activity. In general, their action is to allow waste material to be more effectively washed away.

Oxidizing Agents

Oxidizing agents gain their effectiveness by their ability to transfer ions to microbial protein molecules. If this transfer inactivates a cell enzyme, the effect may be to kill the bacteria. *Hydrogen peroxide* is an example of an agent that releases its oxygen readily. It can have a bacteriocidal effect and also will prevent the growth of anaerobic bacteria.

Halogens are powerful oxidizing agents. They include iodine, chlorine, bromine and fluoride.

Iodine is used primarily as an antiseptic as tincture of iodine (iodine plus alcohol); more recently as a povidone-iodine solution. Iodine solutions have also been used as disinfectants. Iodine has the disadvantage of staining the skin and, if used on large surfaces, the alcohol present in a solution of tincture of iodine may be irritating to the surface. Occasionally, an allergic reaction may result from iodine.

Chlorine is used either as a gas or in liquid form and is most commonly used for a disinfectant as sodium or potassium hypochlorite. Free or available chlorine is released from the solution which combines with water to form hypochloric acid, a potent oxidizing agent. The disadvantage of chlorine agents are their bleaching properties and their strong odors. Chlorine is inactivated by organic matter.

Bromide and fluoride are not generally used as disinfectants because they are toxic in the concentrations required for effectiveness.

Glutaraldehyde

The microbial action of glutaraldehyde is unclear. Although it is thought to react with proteins and enzymes, particularly in an alkaline pH, it does not appear to be inactivated by organic matter. It requires a twenty-minute contact time to be effective against vegetative cells, spores, fungi and some viruses and up to ten hours of contact to be effective against some spores.[15] An alkaline pH is necessary for effective activity, and at this pH, it is stable for no more than fourteen days. Solutions are supplied in two separate containers (one is the alkalinizer) to be combined just before use. It has low toxicity and is non-corrosive. It is relatively expensive and is used primarily for things like lenses and hinged instruments. An example is Cidex™.

Gas Sterilization

Ethylene oxide has been effectively used as a sterilizing agent. It is used in a closed chamber, similar to an autoclave under pressure, and will kill all forms of microorganisms. It penetrates slowly and disperses slowly, requiring a total of about eight hours to sterilize and aerate sufficiently. Ethylene oxide may be toxic to humans, so it must be removed from objects before use. Follow aeration instructions provided with ethylene oxide chamber. It is highly flammable and explosive unless mixed with CO_2. It must be used with care. However, it is very effective for use with moisture-sensitive items and those made of synthetic materials (e.g. catheters) which cannot withstand the temperature and moisture of autoclaving.

Disinfection Procedures

In health care facilities where autoclave and ethylene oxide chambers are available, most urinary drainage supplies can be safely packaged and sterilized. Many items are disposable, used once and discarded. In some hospitals, rehabilitation centers and other health care facilities, patients are taught how to care for their appliances at home, with some items being *disinfected* for reuse. It is highly recommended that if patients are being taught these procedures, they be allowed to practice with *samples* of equipment, *not* those actually in use. The high incidence of potential pathogens present in health care facilities will increase the possibility of nosocomial infections resulting from handling and practicing with used items.

Since after discharge from a health care facility patients may find it financially impossible to use new sterile items daily (e.g. leg bags and tubing), a safe effective method of disinfection is necessary for reuse of equipment. Remember, anything less than sterile increases the danger of infection. An effort should be made to work out the best procedure possible within the limits of the patient's ability, both physical and financial.

Choosing a Method

Included here are a list of supplies frequently used by patients along with suggested *disinfection* methods. It must be remembered that these are all methods meant to *disinfect*, not to *sterilize*, and that equipment treated in this manner should never be considered sterile. Since the composition of manufactured products varies, some items may not withstand the suggested method. It is best to try one item first before deciding on a method.

Item	Disinfection Procedures
Indwelling or suprapubic catheters	Never reuse, discard after use. New catheters should be inserted at least once a month.
Tubing (plastic, etc.)	Use chemical disinfectant, alcohol or boiling. Some types may not withstand boiling.
Tubing (rubber)	Boiling recommended. Chemical solutions frequently affect rubber.
Leg bags (plastic, etc.)	Chemical disinfection or boiling (some types may not withstand boiling).
Leg bags (rubber)	Boiling recommended. Some types may be affected by chemical solutions.
Night jugs or bottles	Chemical disinfection.
Adapters	Boiling or alcohol.
Rubber stoppers, caps, etc.	Boiling or alcohol.
Ostomy Appliances	
Pouches (plastic)	Never reuse. Discard after use.
Pouches (rubber)	Boiling recommended. Some types may be affected by chemical solutions.
Face plates, mounting rings	Alcohol.
Adaptors' plugs, caps	Alcohol.
Catheters for intermittent catheterization	For a sterile catheterization program, discard catheter after use. Do not reuse.

If a less than sterile technique is used, see Chapter VIII. Catheters may be disinfected by boiling or alcohol.

Choosing a Disinfectant

When choosing a disinfecting solution, be sure to read the label carefully. Understand the function of the solution (see "Chemical Disinfectants" in this chapter). Is it a disinfectant or a sanitizer? Some compounds have differing dilution instructions for each. Be sure you use the manufacturer's recommended dilution for *disinfection.*

All solutions should be freshly diluted before use. Do not allow diluted solutions to stand. Discard all solutions after use. Do not reuse them a second day. They may have become inactivated by organic matter, soaps or detergents. If using a compound that is obtained in a powder form, mix only what you will need at one time. Do not mix ahead of time and allow to stand. Some may become inactivated by contaminants and actually support bacterial growth (e.g. quaternary ammonium compounds).

We have found that the phenol compounds work well. However, phenol is irritating to the skin and needs to be rinsed off well. On the other hand, they are less likely to be inactivated by organic matter or residual detergent if washing and rinsing was incomplete. They are relatively inexpensive, do not stain or bleach clothing, and are not excessively corrosive.

The amount of diluted disinfecting solution required will depend to some degree on the size container used. A large container will require more solution. We have found that a plastic shoe box works well, as it will accommodate a leg bag and tubing with a minimum of solution required. Marks placed on the side of the container to indicate 2 quarts, 3 quarts, etc., eliminate the necessity of measuring out the amount of water each time (Fig. XI-1A). Similarly, a small container or cup can be marked with the amount of concentrated disinfectant required (Fig. XI-1B). This will save time when preparing the solution.

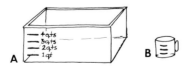

Figure XI-1. Utensils for preparing disinfection solution. A. Plastic container (shoe box) premarked for the volume of disinfection solution needed. B. Small container premarked for the amount of concentrated disinfectant necessary for desired amount of diluted disinfecting solution.

Disinfecting with Chemical Agents

Procedure: The following is a procedure for disinfecting with chemical agents (except alcohol).

1. Put on non-sterile gloves (to protect your hands).
2. Disconnect and separate all parts. Remove straps from leg bag. (They do not need disinfecting but may require washing.)

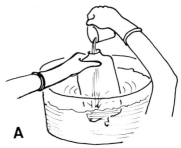

A

Figure XI-2 A–D. Urinary drainage appliance prepared for disinfection.

3. Rinse out gross contamination with water. Discard water properly, as it is contaminated (Fig. XI-2A).

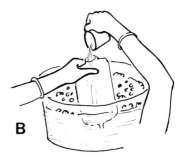

B

4. Wash all items with detergent and water. (All items must be clean before disinfection) (Fig. XI-2B). Discard wash water properly: it is contaminated (Fig. XI-2C).

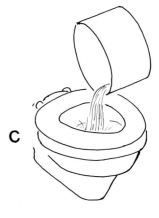

C

5. Rinse out all detergent (Fig. XI-2D). (Some disinfectants are inactivated by detergents. Discard rinse water properly) (Fig. XI-2C).

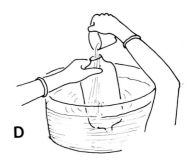

6. Prepare disinfecting solution according to instructions. Read the label carefully (Fig. XI-3A).

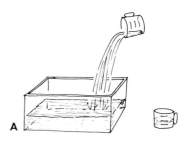

Figure XI-3 A–D. Urinary drainage appliance disinfection. See text.

7. Place items in disinfecting solution. Remove all air bubbles. Be sure all surfaces are exposed to the disinfectant. Put some disinfectant inside leg bag and squeeze out all bubbles. A plastic squeeze bottle or syringe works well for this (Fig. XI-3B). Place tubing in solution so that no air bubbles remain in the tubing. Place one end of tubing in the solution and gradually submerge the remainder, coiling tubing if necessary to fit in container (Fig. XI-3C).

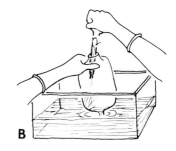

8. Soak for at least thirty minutes. Longer is all right, although some products deteriorate faster with longer soaking (Fig. XI-3D).

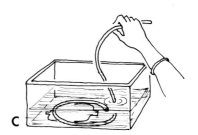

9. Remove items from disinfectant and rinse with boiled water. (Some disinfectants are irritating to the skin and must be rinsed off.) This disinfectant can then be reserved to place in night jug. See step 12.

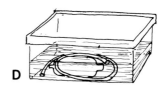

To prepare boiled water: boil water in a covered kettle for thirty minutes and allow it to cool or boil water in a tea kettle (preferably with a covered spout) for thirty minutes and allow to cool (Fig. XI-4).

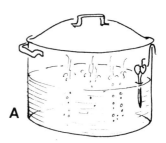

Figure XI-4 A–B. Boiled water prepared. A. Covered kettle. B. Tea-kettle with a covered spout.

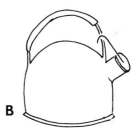

a. To rinse in kettle, remove items from the disinfection solution with a clamp which has been disinfected in alcohol or boiled. Swish items through boiled water to rinse. Allow water to go into tubing and leg bags (Fig. XI-5 A–B). (Do not put hands in boiled water.)

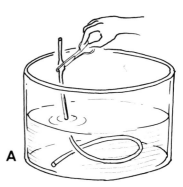

Figure XI-5 A–D. Appliances rinsed with boiled water. A. Tubing rinsed with boiled water in a kettle. B. Bag rinsed with boiled water in a kettle. C. Bag rinsed with cooled boiled water from a teakettle. D. Tubing rinsed with cooled boiled water from a teakettle.

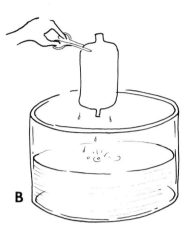

B

b. To rinse with a tea kettle, wipe spout
   to remove any dust particles. Pour
   water through tubing and into leg
   bag. Allow water to rinse outside of
   bag and tubing, also. Be careful *not
   to touch open ends* (Fig. XI-5C–D).
c. If, after rinsing items, disinfectant
   residue still remains, the *outside* can
   be rinsed or washed with tap water.
   Be careful not to contaminate open ends.

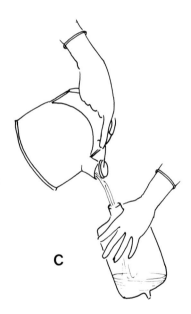

C

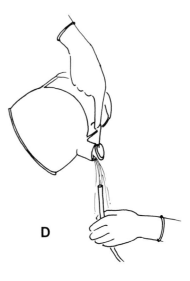

D

10. Hang items to dry if not to be reused immediately. Pull sides of leg bag apart to allow air to enter bag and speed drying (Fig. XI-6). Cover upper open end of leg bag to prevent dust or bacteria dropping into bag (Fig. XI-6).
11. After the bag is dry, cover open ends with sterile gauze pads or alcohol wipes and store in clean place.
12. To disinfect night jug, rinse, wash with detergents, rinse, and fill with disinfectant solution. (The solution from which the leg bag and tubing were removed may be used.) It may be necessary to prepare some additional solution to fill the jug. The solution may remain in the jug until reused. *Discard* the disinfectant. (Do not reuse a second day.) Wipe around the top vigorously with alcohol before replacing the stopper or cap.

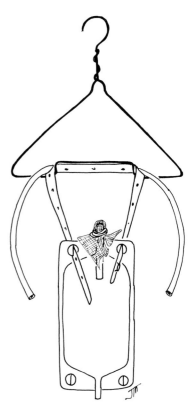

Figure XI-6. Urinary appliances drying after disinfection and rinsing.

Storing Disinfected Equipment

After equipment is dry, cover any open ends with sterile gauze pads or alcohol wipes.

1. Cover ends of tubing with alcohol wipes or sterile gauze pads (Fig. XI-7A).

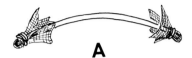

Figure XI-7 A–C. Storing appliances. Open ends covered with sterile gauze squares. A. Tubing. B. Leg Bag. C. Jug.

2. Cover ends of leg bags with disinfected cap, sterile gauze pads or alcohol wipes (Fig. XI-7B).

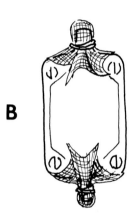

3. Cover top of night jug or bottle (Fig. XI-7C).
4. Store equipment in either a clean towel or in a clean empty container.

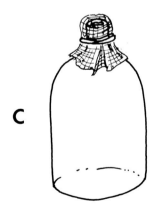

Disinfecting with alcohol

1. Put on non-sterile gloves.
2. Rinse, wash with detergent and rinse all items (see previous "Chemical Disinfection" section).

3. Dry items to be disinfected (excess water will dilute the alcohol).
4. Place items in 70 percent ethyl or isopropyl (rubbing) alcohol. Be sure items are completely submerged (no air bubbles inside tubing, adaptors, etc.).
5. Cover container to prevent alcohol evaporation (Fig. XI-8).
6. Allow items to remain in alcohol until needed (for at least ten minutes).
7. Remove items with a forceps or clamp. Place clamp in alcohol or disinfect it prior to use. Alcohol will evaporate from item rapidly.

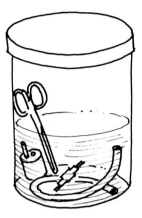

Figure XI-8. Covered containers for 70 percent alcohol used to disinfect some urinary drainage equipment.

Alcohol should be kept covered to avoid evaporation and should be replaced with fresh alcohol at least once a week.

We have found alcohol works well for disinfection of small items (e.g. caps, connectors, stoppers). It is rather expensive to use for large items.

NOTE: If alcohol is to be used for disinfecting catheters used with clean intermittent catheterization program, care must be taken to be sure all the lubricant has been washed off the catheter, that the catheter is clean and dry inside and out before placing in the alcohol, and that the alcohol fills the inside of the catheter (see Chap. XIII, "Disinfection of Reusable Catheters").

Disinfecting by Boiling

Use a covered container that will be large enough to hold all items and contain enough water so as to not boil dry during process.

1. Put on non-sterile gloves.
2. *Rinse,* wash with *detergent* and *rinse* again all items to be boiled (see above "Chemical Disinfection").

3. A forcep or clamp to be used to remove items may be sterilized by boiling or with alcohol. To sterilize by boiling, hang forceps from a wire clamped over the edge of container (Fig. XI-9A).

4. Place items in container. Cover with water. Cover container and bring to a boil. Boil slowly for *thirty minutes*. Keep covered and allow to cool (Fig. XI-9A).

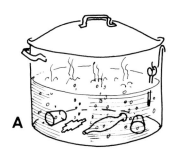

Figure XI-9 A–C. Disinfection by boiling. A. Objects boiling in a covered container. B. Water drained from container after boiling. C. Objects stored in same covered container.

5. If items are to be used soon, they may be left in the water in the container. Keep the container covered. The water may be poured off and items stored in the same covered container (be careful not to touch the inside of the pan or cover) or transferred with disinfected forceps to a boiled covered jar for use at a later time (Fig. XI-9B–C).

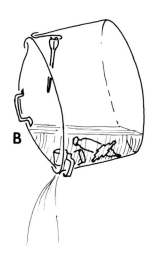

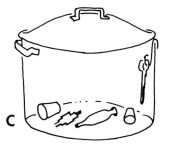

A covered jar can be prepared by placing it in the same kettle and boiling it with other items.

Positioning Urinary Drainage Equipment

1. Urinary drainage equipment should always be kept *below* the level of the bladder or ostomy appliance. At no time should urine be allowed to flow back through the tubing toward the body. Tubing should be in a straight descending line, with no coils, kinks or loops.

2. When moving appliances (e.g. from one side of the bed to the other), clamp off tubing close to body either with forceps or by bending and pinching the tubing. *BE SURE TO UNCLAMP* when move completed (Fig. XI-10).

3. If the patient is using a leg bag, it should be removed from leg and placed on or over edge of bed while patient is lying down (Fig. XI-11).

4. During exercises or range of motion, tubing should be clamped or leg bag removed from leg and placed beside patient (Fig. XI-12).

5. During transportation on stretcher or litter, urine collecting device should be placed over edge of the litter (below body) to allow urine to flow away from body (Fig. XI-13).

6. When the patient is seated in a chair, the collection bag should always be below the level of bladder. Hooks placed under the chair will be an aid (Fig. XI-14).

7. If leg bag is worn, it should be placed below the knee to allow free flow of urine away from the bladder (Fig. XI-15). The leg bag straps should always be placed in such a manner that they lie behind the leg bag. This will allow the bag to pull away from the leg as it fills. If the straps are placed so that they will tighten as the bag fills, this could hinder circulation and cause the foot to swell (Figure XI-16).

8. In a whirlpool or bathtub, the tubing can be clamped off close to the body and drainage bag hung over the edge of the tub. If the patient is to be in this position for a long period of time or has a very small bladder, it may be necessary to raise the patient out of the water periodically, unclamp the tubing and allow bladder to drain (Fig. XI-17).

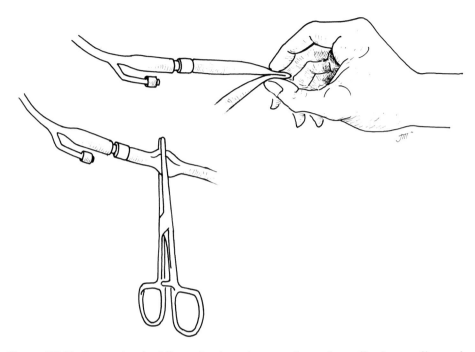

Figure XI-10. Preventing backflow of urine when moving urine collection appliances by clamping off tubing with forceps or by bending and pinching tubing.

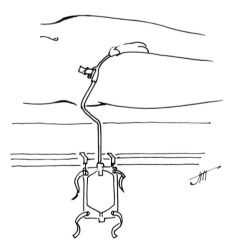

Figure XI-11. Proper positioning of leg bag when patient supine.

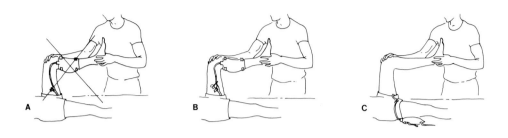

Figure XI-12 A–C. Proper handling of leg bag during activities. A. Incorrect. B. Correct. Tubing clamped. C. Correct. Bag below level of bladder.

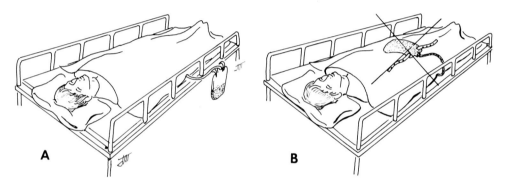

Figure XI-13 A–B. Positioning of urine collection appliance during transport. A. Correct. B. Incorrect.

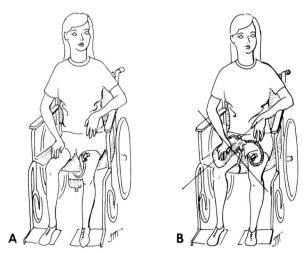

Figure XI-14 A–B. Positioning of urine collection appliances in wheelchair. A. Correct. B. Incorrect.

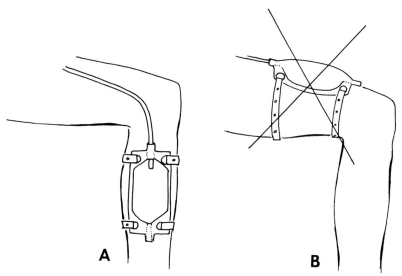

Figure XI-15 A–B. Placement of leg bag. A. Correct. B. Incorrect.

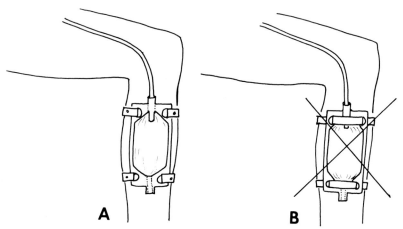

Figure XI-16 A–B. Placement of straps on leg bag. A. Correct. B. Incorrect.

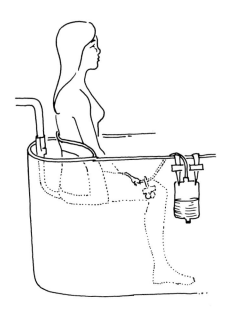

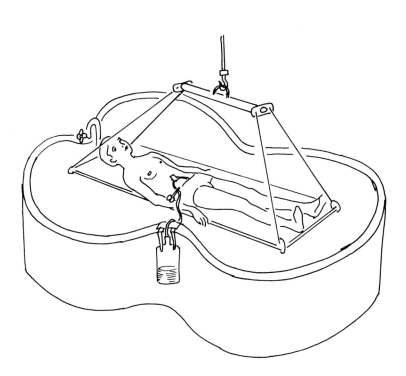

Figure XI-17. Positioning of urinary drainage appliance in whirlpool or tub. A. Seated. B. Supine.

Disconnecting or Emptying Appliances

1. Put on non-sterile gloves (to protect your hands as well as patient). This is particularly important in health care facilities where danger of nosocomial infections is high.
2. To disconnect tubing and appliance, wipe connection site well with alcohol wipes or gauze pad and alcohol before separating. Cover open ends with sterile gauze pad or alcohol wipes (Fig. XI-18).
3. To empty urine collecting device, wipe drainage spout with alcohol wipe or gauze pad and alcohol (Fig. XI-19A). Remove cap or release clamp. Allow urine to drain into a receptacle (Fig. XI-19B). Be careful not to allow urine to splash or spray and contaminate the environment (Fig. XI-19B). Gently tap to remove urine remaining in emptying spout (Fig. XI-19C). Wipe spout with alcohol and reclamp or recap (Fig. XI-19D).

Dispose of urine properly. *Never use same urinal or receptacle for two patients.*

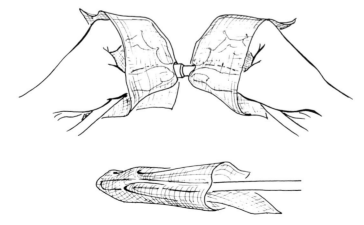

Figure XI-18. Disconnection of urinary appliance and tubing. A. Wipe with alcohol and hold with sterile gauze squares. B. Cover open ends with sterile gauze square.

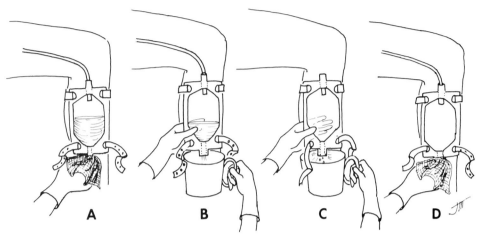

Figure XI-19. Emptying urine collection appliance. A. Wipe emptying spout with alcohol wipe and open spout. B. Drain urine into receptacle. C. Gently tap out urine remaining in spout. D. Wipe spout with alcohol and close.

Supply Kits

One of the most common reasons given by patients for lack of good self-care is the poor availability of supplies and convenient storage space.

A supply kit helps alleviate these problems, both at home and when traveling. A small metal toolbox provides a durable carrying case. The patient can be assisted in outfitting the case with all needed items before discharge from the hospital. A checklist inside the cover will help the patient when replacing used items (Fig. XI-20).

E.N.

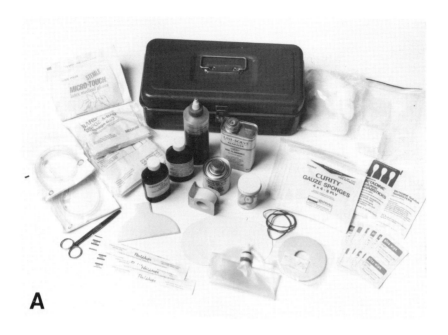

A

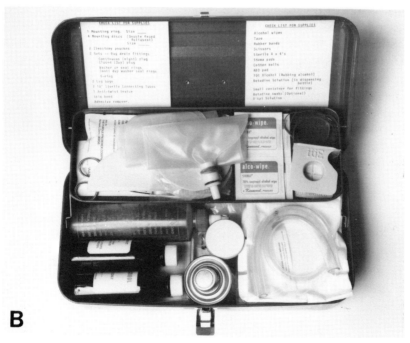

B

Figure XI-20 A–B. Supply kit for patient with supravesical diversion. A. Supplies necessary for care. B. Supplies fitted into a metal "tool box." Lists of supplies placed inside cover.

REFERENCES

1. Bailey, R. R.: Urinary tract Infection — Some recent concepts. *Can Med Assoc 107:*316–330, 1972.
2. Kunin, C.M.: Epidemiology of bacteria and its relation to pyelonephritis. *J Infect Dis 120:*1–11, 1969.
3. Mulholland, S.G., and Bruun, J.N.: A study of hospital urinary tract infections. *J Urol 110:*245–248, 1973.
4. Franzblau, A.H.: Regional differences in patterns of urinary tract infection. *Urol 6:*30–33, 1975.
5. Needham, R.N., Smith, M.M., and Matsen, J.M.: Differences in the bacteriology of intestinal loop urinary diversions. *J Urol 104:*831–833, 1970.
6. Parsons, C.L., Greenspan, C., and Mulholland, S.G.: The primary antibacterial defense mechanism of the bladder. *Invest Urol 13:*72–76, 1975.
7. Donovan, W.H., Stolov, W.C., Clowers, D.E., and Clowers, M.R.: Bacteriuria during intermittent catheterization following spinal cord injury. *Arch Phys Med Rehabil 59:*351–357, 1978.
8. Bulletin: Center for Disease Control, National Nosocomial Infection Study Report. U.S. Dep of Health Education and Welfare. HEW Publication (CDC), No. 80.8257, November, 1979.
9. Garvey, G.: Hospital acquired infections: An approach to the problem. *JAMWA 32:*447–449, 1977.
10. Hardy, P.C., Ederer, G.M., and Matsen, J.M.: Contamination of commercially packaged urinary catheter kits with the pseudomonad EO-1. *N Eng J Med 282:*33–35, 1970.
11. Fierer, J., and Ekstrom, M.: An outbreak of *Providencia stuartii* urinary tract infections. Patients with condom catheters are a reservoir of the bacteria. *JAMA 245:*1553–1555, 1981.
12. Albert, R.K., and Condie, F.: Hand washing patterns in medical intensive-care units. *N Engl J Med 304:*1465–1466, 1981.
13. Maki, D.G., Hennekens, C.H., and Bennett, J.V.: Prevention of catheter-associated urinary tract infection: An additional measure. *JAMA 221:*1270–1271, 1972.
14. Wilson, N.E., Mizer, H.E.: *Microbiology in Patient Care.* 2nd ed. New York, MacMillan, 1974.
15. Russell, A.D., Hugo, W.B., and Ayliffe, G.A.J. (Eds.): *Principles and Practice of Disinfection, Preservation and Sterilization.* Oxford, Blackwell Scientific Publications, 1982.

Chapter XII

URINE CULTURES AND LABORATORY PROCEDURES

URINE CULTURES—WHAT DO THEY MEAN?

To properly identify the microorganisms in a urine specimen and the antibiotic sensitivity pattern, the services of some type of laboratory are required. This may be a sophisticated diagnostic laboratory in a health care facility or a small laboratory in a doctor's office. It is important to understand the services offered, the limitations of these services and the factors that can influence the results in order to obtain culture reports that will be of value.

It is the laboratory's responsibility to promptly and accurately process the specimen and report the results, to maintain good quality control, and to inform the clinician of changes in procedure, rules and regulations. It is the physician's responsibility to be aware of the culture procedures and quality control of the laboratory, to require proper collection, handling and delivery of urine specimens, as well as to understand the factors that can affect the significance of the culture results.

Factors Relating to the Reliability of the Culture Results

Information Supplied on the Request Form

The date and time of culture and method used to obtain the specimen should be stated, as well as a tentative diagnosis if known. Any antibiotics the patient is taking should be listed, as the presence of antibiotics in the urine can influence the rate of growth of any bacteria present. This may necessitate a longer incubation period before final reading.

It is also good to indicate if the person was excessively hydrated in order to obtain the specimen. If the original culture request form is returned to the physician with the culture result, this information is then readily available to the clinician to aid in the interpretation of the culture report.

Method of Obtaining Specimen

The method used to obtain the specimen will vary with the patient. However, one should always try to collect a specimen that will reflect as near as possible the condition within the bladder or urinary conduit, with the least risk to the patient.

The most frequently used methods for obtaining urine specimens are clean catch, catheterization, and aspiration from an indwelling urethral or suprapubic catheter. Specimens obtained from patients with an ileal diversion are obtained by catheterization of the ileal conduit.[1,2]

Time Lapse Between Obtaining Specimen and Culturing

Most microorganisms responsible for urinary tract infections have a rapid growth rate with a doubling time of 20–30 minutes. Bacteria present in an unrefrigerated urine specimen will continue to multiply from the time the specimen was obtained until culturing. Therefore, specimens should be delivered immediately or refrigerated for delivery within the hour.

Specimens to be transported distances should be kept cold (but not frozen) and delivered within an hour from the time obtained.

In addition to the effect of lapsed time on the quantity of organisms present, the relative concentration of organisms present can be affected by delay in culturing.

For example, *E. coli* has a more rapid growth rate and shorter lag phase than many other urinary pathogens and can significantly outgrow other organisms in a period of time.[3]

Reliability of Microbiology Lab and Culture Procedures

The culture procedure used by the laboratory available to you may vary from a simple screening test to a definitive diagnostic procedure. The reports will, therefore, vary from qualitative to specific. Know what you can expect in terms of organism identification and colony counts. Since the type of patients we are concerned with in this discussion frequently have mixed microflora in their urine, often with different sensitivity patterns, culturing procedures that will identify the species of organisms present before and after treatment will be of greater value. Knowing the species of organisms present will also help in identifying sources of infection.

Knowledge of the amount of urine used in the culture procedure will help in evaluating results. For example, if one-tenth of a milliliter of urine is plated, a reported colony count of 1,000 col/ml would mean 100 colonies were present on the culture plate ($100 \times 10 = 1,000$). However, if onethousanth of a milliliter of urine is used, a colony count of 1,000 col/ml would indicate that only one colony (1 × 1,000 = 1,000) was present on the culture plate. One colony could possibly be a contaminant, but it is less likely that 100 colonies would be contaminants.

Standard Culture Procedures: The *streak plate* method, used in many diagnostic microbiology laboratories, consists of streaking a fixed amount of urine onto agar plates with a calibrated loop (e.g. 0.001 ml). Often, two plates are used with different growth media in each to help differentiate species of microorganisms. These plates are incubated at 37° C. The organisms growing on the plates can be counted to determine the colony count and further subcultured to establish species identification and antibiotic sensitivity patterns.

Urine may also be cultured using a *pour* plate method. A specific amount of urine is diluted with a buffer solution. A standard amount of this diluted urine (e.g. 0.1 ml) is added to molten agar poured into a sterile culture plate and incubated. The colonies growing in the media are counted and multiplied by the dilution to obtain the colony count. Colonies may be further subcultured for species identification and antibiotic sensitivity determinations.

Other methods, including automated rapid culturing, chemical, and gas liquid chromatography are currently being developed. Some may prove to be useful in the future for routine diagnostic laboratory use.

Screening Culture Procedure: Simplified urine culture procedures are frequently used as a screening test to determine the presence of bacteriuria in large populations (e.g. school children). They are also frequently used in doctors' offices and small clinics where more definitive procedures are not available. These simplified culture procedures are often used to monitor the urine of patients having a trial off catheter or who are on an intermittent catheterization program. A urine specimen is tested daily with a simple culture procedure, and if that is positive a urine specimen is sent to a diagnostic microbiology lab for a more definitive culture and antibiotic sensitivity tests.

The simplified cultures have the advantage of being inexpensive and easy to perform. They do not require a variety of culture media or elaborate equipment (usually only a small incubator).

Although they will identify the presence or absence of bacteriuria, many screening procedures have the disadvantage of not being able to identify the species of microorganisms present. Some procedures will differentiate between Gram-positive and Gram-negative organisms. Since patients with long-term urinary problems have multiple species of organisms present in their urine, the species would have to be separated and grown in pure culture before antibiotic sensitivity tests can be accurately performed.

There are several different types of culturing procedures available and new ones are being developed. Two examples are given here.

The *filter paper method* involves soaking a precisely sized piece of filter paper in the urine specimens and then gently pressing it on the surface of a small square of culture media. The filter paper is then discarded, the media covered and incubated. The number of organisms growing on the square of media will give an estimate of the number of organisms present. Further subculturing will be required for identification of the organisms and antibiotic sensitivities (example: Testuria®).

Another type of screening method involves the use of a slide coated on each side with different types of growth media. This is referred to as a *dip slide method.* The slide is dipped into a specimen of urine, placed in a storage container and incubated. Bacterial growth on the two types of media are compared and results will partially differentiate the types of organisms present depending upon the types of growth media used on the two sides of the slide. An estimate of colony count can be made from the density of colonies on the slide (example: Uricult®).

Factors Relating to the Significance of the Culture Results

Equally as important as knowing the culture procedure used is an understanding of the factors that can influence the colony count. In 1956, Kass[4] reported on the use of colony counts to differentiate between significant and non-significant culture results.

A colony count of 100,000 or greater per milliliter soon was accepted as the concentration used to identify true infection. More recent studies have shown that infections can result in lower bacterial counts.[5-7] This is particularly true in patients with long-term genitourinary problems and chronic pyelonephritis[7-9] and for patients with ileal diversions.[10]

The concentration of organisms present in the urine can depend on: bacterial growth rate; hydration; time of day specimen is obtained; cohesion or adhesion of infected material; surgical procedures or congenital abnormalities; reflux and residual urine; chronic pyelonephritis; and anaerobic, phage, L-forms and fastidious organisms.

Bacterial Growth Rate

The growth rate may be slowed down by the presence of antibiotics or bacteriostatic elements in the urine. Slower-growing species may be "overgrown" on the culture plates.

Hydration

The flow rate and the volume of the system will affect the concentration of organisms present, as well as the length of time that the infected urine remains in the bladder. An increase in the flow of fresh urine into a small capacity bladder or one being constantly drained with an indwelling catheter or an ileal conduit will have a greater dilution effect than the same amount of fresh urine into a large volume.

The change that can result from hydration and the shortening of the time that urine remains in the bladder is sufficient to result in a colony count below 100,000 col/ml, further demonstrating the danger of using a specific colony count to determine the significance of bacteriuria.[11]

Time of Day Specimen is Obtained

Since bacteria remaining in the bladder overnight will have had more time to multiply, they will be present in higher concentration than if they remained in the bladder for only a short time. Pryles reported on this effect in 1971[6], showing that colony counts can drop from 10^8 at 7 A.M. to 10^3 at 6 P.M.

Bacteria will frequently accumulate in certain areas of the urinary tract, such as diverticula, trabecular pockets and saccules, and be released intermittently into urine, thereby causing fluctuation in colony counts.[12] Changing the position of a patient can alter the colony count by emptying urine from stagnant pools.

Cohesion or Adhesion of Infected Material

Some bacteria such as *E. coli* can grow in sheets attached to mucus or the bladder wall. When these sheets are released into the urine, they will greatly alter the colony count.

Surgical Procedures or Congenital Abnormalities

Such condition can permit pooling of urine in areas and contribute to unequal washout.

Reflux and Residual Urine

Reflux and high residuals prevent complete emptying of the bladder, thus decreasing "washout" effect of urine flow leading to higher colony counts.

Chronic Pyelonephritis

Patients with chronic pyelonephritis may have very low colony counts, as only a few bacteria at a time may be released into the urine.[7,8] The length of time this urine then remains in the bladder will influence the number of organisms reported in the culture result.

Anaerobic, Phage, L-forms and Fastidious Organisms

Several types of microorganisms that do not grow under routine culturing procedures are being recognized as the etiology of some urinary tract infections.[13] Research is being conducted to develop special culturing procedures, but these are not routinely available. We should keep in mind, though, that a patient may have a urinary tract infection, even if repeated urine cultures show no growth. Anaerobes, phages, L-forms and fastidious organisms are discussed in Chapter III.

Summary

We have described some examples of factors that can lead to variations in colony counts to help us to understand the importance of not relying entirely on colony counts when evaluating the significance of a urine culture or the effectiveness of therapy.

Each culture result requires careful evaluation and clinical judgement. Knowledge of the mode of drainage in use and the method of specimen collection, as well as the other factors such as time of day, degree of hydration and anatomical variations, will modify the interpretation of culture results.

Positive urine cultures, regardless of colony counts, do not necessarily indicate the presence of urinary tract infections. However, since many of the patients with long-term urinary problems do not develop or display the classical symptoms of a urinary tract infection, be alert to the possibility of infection. The decision of when to treat is indeed a challenge to the clinician.

In order to obtain the most help from the laboratory, it is important to supply it with properly obtained and promptly delivered specimens and provide the necessary information to enable the personnel to use correct culturing procedures.

Be aware of the limitations of the culturing procedure used and be free to ask questions.

Urine cultures from patients with long-term genitourinary tract problems may differ from cultures from the general population, frequently containing multiple species of microorganisms, lower colony counts, and having different sensitivity patterns. An understanding of these factors should help the clinician in the management and care of this type of patient.

ANTIBIOTIC SENSITIVITY DETERMINATIONS

Multiple species of microorganisms frequently are present in cultures from patients with long-term urinary problems, and the sensitivity patterns for these organisms often differ from that of organisms isolated from the general population. This is probably due to the frequent use of antibiotics, which can lead to the emergence of resistant strains, either through selection, mutation or R-factor transfer.[7] Obtaining sensitivity test results will aid in the selection of the most effective antimicrobial methods.

The Bauer-Kirby disc and the tube dilution procedures are methods frequently used for antimicrobial susceptibility testing. Results from these procedures are usually reported as sensitive, intermediate or resistant. The determinations are based primarily on the antimicrobial concentrations achieved in the serum by using the "usual" doses as listed on the package inserts. There are many conditions that can affect the results of this test.

In recent years, microdilution determinations have been developed that permit a simple accurate determination of the minimum inhibitory concentration (MIC) value for test organisms against many microbial agents.

MIC is the lowest concentration of an antimicrobial agent which will inhibit the in vitro growth of the tested organism. Results of the microdilution tests are usually reported in mcg/ml. MIC values are more correctly related to the in vivo inhibitory levels achievable with various doses and rates of administration, and more directly applicable to concentrations achievable at the site of infection. These facts are particularly important in the treatment of urinary tract infections, as the concentrations of some antimicrobials, such as aminoglycosides, may be much greater in the urine than in the serum. In vitro values do not always apply in vivo, as other factors may influence the effectiveness of an antibiotic.

LOCALIZATION PROCEDURES

Localization procedures are tests that will help to identify the site of a urinary tract infection. Since the treatment and management of upper tract infections may differ from that of lower tract infections, a reliable localization test would be an aid to the clinician.

Included here is a brief description of three procedures that have been shown to be of some value in the localization of the site of infection.

The Fairley Bladder Washout

The Fairley Bladder Washout test is probably the most accurate localization test to date, although in males it may not differentiate upper tract infection from prostatitis.[14] The test consists of a series of urine cultures taken before, during and after a bladder washout procedure. An antibiotic solution (usually neomycin) is instilled into the bladder for 30–45 minutes. This is followed by a continuous flushing of the bladder with sterile saline. Results of the cultures taken are compared. A positive culture prior to the antibiotic instillation and bladder washout, and continued positive cultures after neomycin instillation and during and after subsequent saline washout, are indications of upper tract infection because they show that bacteria are continually being discharged into the urine by the kidneys. If the urine cultures show no growth after neomycin instillation and after bladder washout, the infection is believed to have its origin in the bladder only. Unfortunately, this procedure is time consuming and not without some risk to the patient. Consequently, it is not performed on a routine basis.

Antibody-Coated Bacteria Determinations

In 1974, Thomas and co-workers[15] reported a test that was said to differentiate between upper and lower tract infections. This test is based on the concept that bacterial invasion of the kidney stimulates production of antibodies which cling to the surface of the bacteria. It was hypothesized that when the infection is in the bladder, no antibodies are produced and the bacteria will not be coated. The presence of antibodies on the surface of the bacteria is demonstrated by an immunofluorescent procedure. Later studies[16] have demonstrated that antibodies may also be produced if bacteria have invaded the bladder wall or prostatic tissue, even though they have not reached the kidneys. It is now recognized that the value of the test is not so much to identify upper or lower tract infection but to determine that tissue invasion by bacteria has taken place. This information should be of value to clinicians in planning treatment. Careful quality control of the collection of specimen and the procedure is important to obtain reliable results. Consistency in establishing criteria to differentiate between a positive and negative test would be helpful in standardizing the procedure.

To date, this procedure is not available in many diagnostic laboratories.

Lactic Dehydrogenase Determinations

Studies by Carvajal and co-workers[17] and others[18,19] have suggested that the measurement of lactic dehydrogenase (LD) in the urine of infants and children can be an aid in identifying the site of infection. Preliminary results from our research suggests that this determination will be of value in adults.[20]

Lactic dehydrogenase is a key glycolytic enzyme. It is almost completely cytoplasmic in origin and composed of five isoenzymes. The quantitative distribution of the five LD isoenzymes is different in various body fluids and tissues and is characteristic for each source. Changes in these patterns have been noted following infection, injury or abnormal metabolic activity.

Investigators have found an increase in urinary LD and an increase in enzyme fractions LD4 and LD5 in children who have pyelonephritis as compared to children with cystitis.

Our study population was composed of adult patients with spinal cord lesions. We found that 81 percent demonstrated changes in lactic dehydrogenase enzyme patterns consistent with bladder or kidney tissue damage. These changes were not always related to bacterial infection. Evidence of tissue damage occurred more frequently in the absence of infection in those patients using external catheters, intermittent catheterization or who were appliance free than in those patients using indwelling urethral or suprapubic catheters.[20] Perhaps this indicates tissue damage due to overdistention.

PROCEDURES FOR OBTAINING URINE SPECIMEN FOR CULTURES

General Information

1. *Reliable results require:* proper collection, prompt delivery to laboratory or refrigeration for delivery within one hour.
2. *Carefully filled out request slips:* Indicate if patient is on antibiotics. Indicate if patient is excessively hydrated. State time of day specimen collected. Include other factors that could affect culture results.
3. *Specimen collection:* Collect specimens that will reflect as much as possible the conditions within the bladder or ileal conduit. Follow appropriate procedures for specimen collection.
4. *BEFORE OBTAINING ANY URINE SPECIMEN FOR CULTURE, WASH HANDS VIGOROUSLY AND PUT ON CLEAN, NON-STERILE GLOVES.*
5. Inquire if the patient is allergic to povidone-iodine.

Clean Catch Specimens

The clean catch method cannot be used when the patient is too obese to clean properly, too ill or immobilized, or cannot void spontaneously. It is a difficult method to use with newborns or infants.

Ambulatory patient (specimen collection with or without assistance as determined by nurse or physician)

Women:

1. Spread labia and hold while cleansing area (Fig. XII-1). Wash slowly with detergent and water three times with rayon balls or absorbent pads. Wipe front toward back. Rinse with tap water.

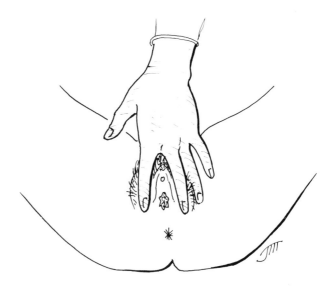

Figure XII-1. Labia separated with fingers to aid in obtaining uncontaminated clean-catch urine specimens.

2. Wipe with povidone-iodine solution or swabs three times front to back. (If patient is allergic to povidone-iodine, omit this step and repeat wash step.)
3. Hold labia apart and pass urine and discard first portion (approx. 10 ml).
4. Pass midstream urine and collect in sterile container. Cover.
5. Wash and rinse perineal area to remove povidone-iodine.

Men:

1. Wash penis three times with detergent and water, retracting foreskin, if not circumcised. Rinse.
2. Wipe meatus and shaft of penis with povidone-iodine solution or swabs. (If patient allergic to povidone-iodine, omit this step and repeat wash step.)

3. Void small amount (approximately 10 ml) and discard.
4. Void midstream into sterile container and cover.
5. Wash and rinse penis to remove povidone-iodine.

Bedridden Patient

Women — Assisted:

1. Place pad under patient and proceed as above for ambulatory patient.

Men — Assisted: Proceed as above for ambulatory men.

Catheterizated Specimens

Catheterization for urine specimens is not generally recommended as a routine method. Use if patient is catheterized for other procedure, unable to void, or markedly obese. Catheterization is also used for women with redundant labia.

1. Use aseptic technique to catheterize patient (see Chap. V, "Catheterization Procedures").
2. Allow urine to flow from end of sterile catheter.
3. Discard first few ml.
4. Collect next urine in sterile container and cover.

Suprapubic Aspiration

Suprapubic aspiration is sometimes used for cultures from newborns and infants, especially girls. Procedures must be performed by physician.

Specimens from Patients with Indwelling Urethral or Suprapubic Catheters

Closed Method (Fig. XII-2)

A closed method is recommended, since it avoids the danger of contamination when the catheter-tubing union is separated. Newer types of solid silicone catheters do not recover from needle punctures, so do not use this method with those catheters. Teflon or silicone-*coated* catheters will recover from needle puncture.

1. Clamp catheter above the catheter-tubing union (Fig. XII-2).
2. Vigorously wipe the catheter-tubing union with alcohol wipes or 70 percent alcohol and sterile gauze pads.

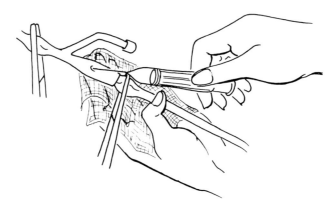

Figure XII-2. Closed method for obtaining urine specimens from a catheter for culture or urinalysis. See text.

3. Place sterile gauze pad under catheter-tubing union (to be used to hold catheter).
4. Allow any urine in adapter or tubing just below the catheter-tubing union to flow down the tubing and then clamp the tubing as close as possible to end of catheter. This will prevent aspirating urine from the tubing for specimen.
5. Using a sterile 24-gauge needle and syringe, insert needle into the flared end of the catheter at a slant, being careful not to puncture channel used to inflate balloon.
6. Release clamp above point of needle insertion (leave clamped below) and aspirate urine specimen.
7. Withdraw needle from catheter, wipe site of puncture with alcohol and remove clamp.
8. Transfer specimen to sterile container.

NOTE: *BE SURE TO UNCLAMP CATHETER AFTER SPECIMEN HAS BEEN OBTAINED.*

Open Method (Fig. XII-3)

An open method should be used if the patient is using a solid silicone catheter or if the catheter-tubing union is being separated for some reason (e.g. changing from leg bag to night drainage system).

1. Clamp catheter above catheter-tubing union.
2. Vigorously wipe catheter-tubing union with alcohol wipes or 70 percent alcohol and sterile gauze pad. Be sure to wipe the end of the catheter.

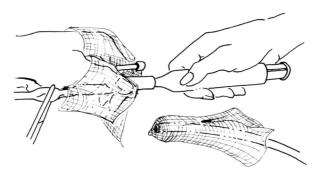

Figure XII-3. Open method for obtaining urine specimens from a catheter for culture or urinalysis. See text.

3. Separate the catheter-tubing union — cover the open end of the tubing with sterile gauze pad.
4. Using a catheter-tipped syringe, unclamp catheter and slowly withdraw urine (Fig. XII-3). If urine is allowed to run directly from the catheter into a sterile container, care must be taken to be sure the urine does not run back along the outside of the catheter before flowing into the container.
5. Transfer the specimen to a sterile container and cover.
6. Wipe end of catheter and tubing with alcohol and reconnect.

Specimens from Patients Using External Catheters

Before beginning, ask patient if his bladder can be triggered to empty and if he can do this himself or needs assistance. Inquire which position the patient should be placed in to most readily trigger bladder (e.g. seated, supine or side).

1. Place patient in proper position.
2. Wash hands and put on non-sterile gloves.
3. Expose perineal area and drape area with waterproof pad and/or towel.
4. Remove external catheter.
5. Wash penis and the perineal area, retracting foreskin, if not circumcised. Repeat washing procedure three times with detergent and water.
6. Wipe meatus and shaft of penis three times with povidone-iodine solution or swabs. If patient is allergic to povidone-iodine, omit this step and repeat wash step.
7. Place non-sterile receptacle under penis to collect first portion of urine.

8. Trigger bladder, using technique patient describes as best (e.g. tapping).
9. When urine begins to flow, allow small amount (approximately 10 ml) to pass into non-sterile container.
10. Collect midstream specimen in sterile container; cover immediately.
11. Wash penis to remove povidone-iodine, rinse and dry.
12. Replace external catheter.

Specimens from Patients with Urinary Diversions

Obtaining urine specimens of uncontaminated urine for cultures from patients with urinary diversion is difficult, requiring meticulous technique to avoid introduction of organisms from the stoma or portions of the loop contiguous to it. Bishop[10] in 1971 devised a method using a catheter with a metal sleeve. Later, Spence, Ireland and Cass[21] developed a telescoping double lumen catheter which avoids the use of an inflexible object and provides a reliable method for obtaining a specimen for culture. This type of catheter can be made up from a No. 16 French whistle-tipped catheter and a No. 8 polyethylene infant feeding tube or it can be obtained already prepared in a sterile package (e.g. Tele-Cath™). The whistle-tipped catheter is cut approximately one inch shorter than the feeding tube. The feeding tube is then inserted into the whistle-tipped catheter (Fig. XII-4). The unit is packaged and gas sterilized. Telescoping catheters are highly recommended, however, if necessary, a Fr. 16 catheter may be used.

Procedures for Double Lumen Catheterization

Supplies Needed

Sterile:

> Catheter kit
> Double lumen catheter
> Syringe (10 or 12 cc)
> Gloves
> Forceps
> Specimen container
> Gauze pads

Non-Sterile:

> Absorbent pads
> pH paper
> Razor or scissor

8 infant feeding tube

16 French whistle tip catheter

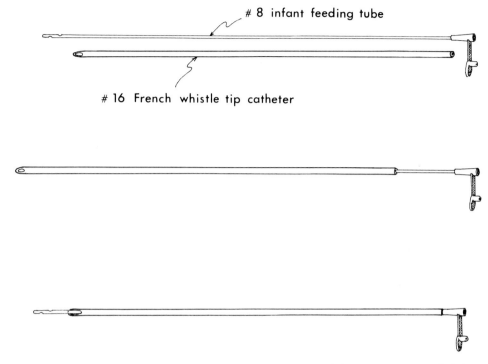

Figure XII-4. A telescopic double lumen catheter constructed from a No. 8 French infant feeding tube and a No. 16 French whistle tip catheter.

Waterproof pad
Soap and water
Adhesive remover
Towel

Procedure

1. Obtain all materials needed.
2. Wash hands and put on non-sterile gloves.
3. Open catheter kit. Use wrapper as sterile field.
4. Place double lumen catheter, sterile syringe and sterile forceps on sterile field. Do not contaminate items.
5. Place piece of pH paper on gauze pad. It is recommended that the pH be determined when a urine specimen is obtained for culture.
6. Place waterproof pad under patient and pad patient with absorbent pads.
7. Drain appliance and remove from patient, using adhesive remover. (Ask patient first if he is sensitive to adhesive remover.)

8. Clean all adhesive from stoma area.
9. If there are hairs growing in the site of mounting disc, these should be removed with a razor or scissors. This will make cleansing easier and provide for better adhesion of mounting disc.
10. Put on sterile gloves.
11. Pour povidone-iodine solution over rayon balls; reserve small amount to pour over stoma.
12. Cleanse stoma area with rayon balls; hold with forceps (supplied with kit).
13. Place sterile drape on patient around stoma.
14. Pour remaining povidone-iodine solution on stoma to insure solution reaching folds in stoma.
15. Place lubricant on tip of catheter.
16. Test catheter to be sure feeding tube goes through end. Close end of feeding tube.
17. Wait for urine flow to wash povidone-iodine solution from stoma and to permit accurate residual measurement.
18. Insert catheter through stoma, using second sterile forceps. (Be sure feeding tube is retracted.) It is sometimes necessary to wait for conduit to relax to allow passage of catheter.
19. After catheter is well within conduit (approx. $3\frac{1}{2}$ inches), insert feeding tube into catheter.
20. Withdraw urine with sterile syringe. (Have assistant do this, if available.) You may have to wait for urine to form.
21. Transfer urine to sterile culture container. Reserve drop for pH paper.
22. Determine pH and record along with residual volume.
23. Wash stoma area and dry.
24. Replace appliance.
25. Send culture specimen directly to microbiology laboratory or refrigerate for delivery within the hour.

NOTE: Careful observation should be made of the stoma when the ostomy appliance is removed to check for areas of irritation, hyperplasia and dermatitis. It is important to wait for urine to flow before inserting the catheter to allow urine to flush off the povidone-iodine solution and to give an accurate measure of conduit residuals. Large residuals should be reported to the physician. An ileal conduit usually contains about 10 cc of urine, a colon or sigmoid conduit slightly more.

An illustrated manual, *Double Lumen Catheterization of the Ileal Conduit,* is available from the Department of Physical Medicine and Rehabilitation,

Box 156 Mayo, University of Minnesota Hospitals, 420 Delaware Street S.E., Minneapolis, MN 55455.

Care of Specimen

1. Use sterile container and be careful not to contaminate when opening and closing container.
2. Replace cover firmly.
3. Attach request forms and labels to container.
4. Deliver promptly or refrigerate for delivery within one hour.

E.N.

REFERENCES

1. Spence, B., Stewart, W., and Cass, A.S.: Use of a double lumen catheter to determine bacteriuria in intestinal loop diversion in children. *J Urol 108:*800, 1972.
2. Newman, E., and Price, M.: *Double Lumen Catheterization of the Ileal Conduit Manual.* Department PM&R, University of Minnesota Hospitals, 1974.
3. Anderson, J.D., Eftekhar, F., Aird, M.Y., and Hammond, J.: Role of bacterial growth rates in the epidemiology and pathogenesis of urinary tract infections in women. *J Clin Micro 10:*766–771 (Dec) 1979.
4. Kass, E.H.: Asymptomatic infections of the urinary tract. *Trans Assoc Am Physicians 67:*56–64, 1956.
5. Motzkin, D.: The bacteriological diagnosis and treatment of urinary tract infection. *J Urol 107:*454–457, 1972.
6. Pryles, C.V., and Lustik, B.: Laboratory diagnosis of urinary tract infection. *Pediatr Clin North Am 18:*233–244, 1971.
7. Stamey, T.A.: *Pathogenesis and Treatment of Urinary Tract Infections.* Baltimore/London, Williams and Wilkins, 1980.
8. Effersøe, P., and Jensen, E.: Urinary tract infection versus bacterial contamination quantitative study. *Lancet 1:*1342–1343, 1963.
9. Seneca, H., and Peer, P.: Clinical laboratory diagnosis of urinary tract infection. *J Urol 94:*78–81, 1965.
10. Bishop, R.F., Smith, E.D., and Gracy, M.: Bacterial flora of urine from ileal conduit. *J Urol 105:*452–455, 1971.
11. Friedman, S.A., and Gladstone, J.L.: The effects of hydration and bladder incubation time on urine colony counts. *J Urol 105:*428–432 (Mar) 1971.
12. O'Grady, F., Path, M.C., and Cattell, W.R.: Kinetics of urinary tract infection. 1. Upper urinary tract infection. *Br J Urol 38:*149–155 (Mar 14) 1966.
13. Martin, W.J., and Segura, J.W.: Urinary tract infections due to anaerobic bacteria. In Belaws, A., DeHaan, R.M., Dowell, V.R., Jr., Guze, L.B. (Eds.): *Anaerobic Bacteria — Role in Disease.* Springfield, Charles C Thomas, Publisher, 1974. (International Conference on Anaerobic Bacteria Center for Disease Control, 1972.)
14. Fairley, K.F., Carson, N.E., Gutch, R.C., Leighton, P., Grounds, D.D., Laird, E.C., McCallum, P.H.G., Sleeman, R.L., and O'Keefe, C.M.: Site of infection in acute urinary tract infection in general practice. *Lancet 3:*615–618, 1971.

15. Thomas, V., Shelokov, A., and Forland, M.: Antibody coated bacteria in the urine and the site of urinary tract infection. *N Engl J Med 290*:588–590, 1974.
16. Jones, S.R.: Prostatitis as cause of antibody-coated bacteria in urine. (Letter) *N Engl J Med 291*:365, 1974.
17. Carvajal, H.F., Passey, R.B., Berger, M., Travis, L.B., and Lorentz, W.B.: Urinary lactic dehydrogenase isoenzyme 5 in the differential diagnosis of kidney and bladder infections. *Kidney Int 8*:176–184, 1975.
18. Lorentz, W.B., and Resnik, M.J.: Comparison of urinary lactic dehydrogenase with antibody coated bacteria in the urine sediment as means of localizing the site of urinary tract infections. *Pediatrics 64*:672–677, 1977.
19. Devaskar, U., and Montgomery, W.: Urinary lactic dehydrogenase isoenzymes IV and V in the differential diagnosis of cystitis and pyelonephritis. *J Ped 93*:789–91, 1978.
20. Newman, E., Ibrahim, G., and Price, M.: Urine lactic dehydrogenase—An aid in the management of patients with spinal cord injury. *Int Rehabil Med 6*:170–172, 1984.
21. Spence, B., Ireland, G.W., and Cass, A.S.: Bacteriuria in intestinal loop diversion in children. *J Urol 106*:780–781, 1971.

Chapter XIII

PHARMACOLOGICAL TREATMENT OF URINARY TRACT INFECTIONS

Treatment of urinary tract infections falls into three categories: preventive or prophylactic, suppressive, and active.

PREVENTION

The most important component of urinary tract infection prevention is a decisive plan to prevent access of bacteria to the bladder together with the use of fluids to wash out organisms which may have gained access. The urine should be kept acid so that most bacteria will not reproduce freely. It is helpful to limit the use of alkalinizing foods and encourage the use of acidifying foods (See Appendix). Fortunately, with proper diet, the uninfected urine is usually acid, but sometimes acidifying drugs must be used, most commonly ascorbic acid and ammonium chloride. The former does not always accomplish its goal and with occasional individuals will lead to the precipitation of oxylate crystals, which not only can irritate the bladder mucosa sufficiently to produce hematuria but can also cause stones. Ammonium chloride must be carefully monitored, since it can alter the body's acid-base balance with resultant acidosis.

Methenamine compounds (Mandelamine, Hiprex) have long been used for prophylaxis and have experienced waxing and waning of popularity. Their sterilizing ability depends upon the release of formaldehyde in the presence of an acid pH.[1]

While occasionally, small doses of sulfonamides (Gantrisin®, Gantanol®) or nitrofurantoin (Macrodantin®) are used for prevention of infection. Such medications are usually reserved for suppression or eradication of bacterial growth.

SUPPRESSION

Suppressive treatment is aimed at keeping the concentrations of bacteria below the level at which they can inflame the bladder lining, invade the bladder wall, gain access to the bloodstream or be carried to the kidneys by reflux. Small doses of sulfonamides or nitrofurantoin are often used for this purpose.

ACTIVE TREATMENT

Active treatment is the vigorous attempt to eradicate infection. Although expense to the patient and ease of administration are important, the primary consideration is the selection of the drug which will most efficiently eradicate the organism with the least possibility of increasing the patient's morbidity. There are many classes of antibacterials[2] and the choice is usually made through antibiotic sensitivity studies, although sometimes the severity of the disease may demand the beginning of treatment before the studies can be completed. The most frequently used groups of antibiotics are sulfonamides, trimethoprim, penicillins, tetracyclines, nitrofurantoins, nalidixic acid, cephalosporins and aminoglycosides.

Sulfonamides

Sulfonamides are bacteriostatic agents often effective against *E. coli, Klebsiella, Enterobacter, Staphylococcus aureus,* and *Proteus.* Because the drugs have been used for many years, a large number of strains have become resistant to the "sulfa" drugs.

Sulfonamides can be given either orally or parenterally. When used orally, they should be taken on an empty stomach with a full glass of water.

Allergy to one sulfonamide generally carries over to all others and also to furosemide (Lasix®), thiazides (Diuril®, Enduron®), glaucoma medications, and many other medications incorporating "sulf" or "amide" in their generic names.

Sulfonamide action is inhibited by the presence of para-aminobenzoic acid (PABA), and the-caine type local anesthetic agents as well as by pus or tissue fluids. They should not be given with oral anticoagulants such as warfarin (Coumadin®) and dicumarol or with oral antidiabetic medications (Diabinase®, Orinase®), methenamine products (Mandelamine, Hiprex), the pencillins, or the anti-gout drug sulfinpyrazone (Antiurane®). They should be used cautiously in the presence of decreased liver function, decreased kidney function or porphyria.

Unpleasant side effects which should be reported to the physician are nausea and vomiting, diarrhea, itching, rash and sensitivity to sunlight. An uncommon but serious complication is the development of blood dyscrasia. Consequently, all long-term administration of sulfonamides should be monitored by periodic blood counts. Although modern sulfonamides are more soluble than their predecessors, it is wise to keep the urine slightly alkaline to discourage crystal formation, especially with the doses necessary for active treatment.

Trimethoprim

Trimethoprim (Proloprim®, Trimpex®) is a bacteriostatic medication which is most often given concurrently with a sulfonamide (Bactrim™) because of their synergistic action upon *E. coli, Proteus, Klebsiella,* and some *Staphylococcus* species. Neither is effective against *Pseudomonas.* It is given orally, preferably on an empty stomach.

Allergic reactions have not been notable but, as the medication is longer in use, may become more frequent.

An adverse effect may be interference with the metabolism of folic acid, in which case a supplement may be indicated.

Other side reactions are headaches, skin rash, unusual taste in the mouth, itching or, more rarely, methemoglobinemia or anemia.

Penicillins

The penicillin group is bactericidal and is most effective with rapidly growing organisms.

Penicillins can be used parenterally but are usually given orally with a full glass of water on an empty stomach. Penicillin G should not be given with fruit juice.

As with sulfonamides, the penicillins have been used for many years so that considerable bacterial resistance has developed increasing the necessity for antibiotic sensitivity determination.

Penicillin allergy is common and can be fatal. There is often cross sensitivity with other penicillins, cephalosporins (Keflex®), griseofulvin (Fulvicin®, Grifulvin®) and penicillamine. Sensitivity may develop to-caine type local anaesthetics used with injectable penicillin.

Penicillin should not be given with bacteriostatic drugs such as the sulfonamides or tetracyclines. It should not be given with the anti-diarrheals which slow peristalsis (opiates, Lomotil®), because the delay in passage of intestinal contents may irritate the bowel mucosa as well as inhibit intestinal flora thus favoring pseudomembranous colitis.

Users of oral contraceptives should be warned that penicillin can significantly decrease the effectiveness of the contraceptive, disrupting the menstrual cycle and increasing the risk of pregnancy.

Concurrent use of neomycin can cause malabsorption of penicillin.

Tetracyclines

The tetracyclines are bacteriostatic drugs effective with *E. coli, Klebsiella, Enterobacter, Acinetobacter* and *Streptococcus.*

Tetracyclines can be given parenterally but are usually taken orally with a full glass of water on an empty stomach. In the presence of gastric distress, they can be given with food, but dairy products must be avoided. They should not be given at the same time as antacids, iron products or vitamins.

Allergy to one tetracycline is usually carried over to the others. Patients may also become sensitized to the-caine type anaesthetics included in intramuscular injections.

A distressing side effect is the inhibition of skeletal growth in the fetus and the discoloration of teeth and hypoplasia of enamel during the formative periods. Hence, tetracyclines should not be given during pregnancy or to young children. Other side effects are nausea and vomiting, diarrhea, sensitivity to sunlight, genital and anal itching and dark coloration of the tongue.

Nitrofurantoins

Nitrofurantoin (Furadantin®, Macrodantin) is a useful antibacterial which is excreted almost entirely by the kidneys. It is both bacteriostatic and bactericidal, depending on its concentration. It is usually effective against *E. coli,* enterococci, *Staphylococcus aureus, Klebsiella, Enterobacter,* and *Proteus.* It should be taken orally with food or milk.

Allergic reactions to one form usually occur in other forms.

Nitrofurantoin causes a yellow or brownish color in the urine. The oral suspension can temporarily color the teeth orange. This can be minimized by rinsing or brushing. Mild side effects are nausea, vomiting, or diarrhea. A less common but more serious complication is allergic penumonitis accompanied by fever. Prolonged administration can result in neuropathy.

Nitrofurantoin should not be given concurrently with nalidixic acid (NegGram®), probenacid or sulfinpyrazone (Anturan®).

Naladixic Acid

Nalidixic acid (NegGram) is a bactericidal medication which affects most Gram-negative organisms except *Pseudomonas.* These include *E. coli, Proteus, Klebsiella,* and *Enterobacter.*

It is given orally with a full glass of water on an empty stomach. If gastric irritation occurs, it can be taken with foods.

There may be cross allergy between nalidixic acid and cinoxacin (Cinobac®).

It should not be given concurrently with nitrofurantoin since the two are antagonistic. It should not be given with oral anticoagulants such as dicumarol and warfarin (Coumadin) because it decreases their effectiveness.

Nalidixic acid should not be used in the presence of central nervous system damage, severe cerebral arteriosclerosis, convulsive disorders, or liver or kidney impairment.

Side effects are blurred vision, change in color vision, double vision, sensitivity to glare, unusual tiredness because of blood dyscrasia, jaundice, abdominal cramps, diarrhea, nausea and vomiting, itching, rash, dizzyness and drowsiness.

Administration should not be longer than two weeks without close supervision by the physician.

Cephalosporins

Cephalosporins are bactericidal drugs of the beta lactam group. They are generally described in three "generations" based on time of discovery and the bacteria which they affect.

Some cephalosporins can only be administered parenterally, some orally, while many can be given by both routes. With oral dosage, they can be taken either with or without food. Alcohol should be avoided during and for several days following cefamandole (Mandol®) administration.

There are cross allergies between the cephalosporins and penicillin, penicillin derivatives and penicillamine.

Cephalosporins should not be given concurrently with aminoglycosides (Garamycin®, Amikacin), ethocrynic acid (Edecrin®), furosemide (Lasix) or polymixin because of the increased potential for neuro-, oto-, or nephrotoxicity.

Mild side effects are nausea and vomiting, abdominal cramps, and diarrhea. More serious are unusual thirst, unusual tiredness, and weight loss due to pseudomembranous colitis.

First-generation cephalosporins include cephadroxil (Ultrocef™), cefazolin (Ancef®), cefalexin (Keflex), cefalothin (Ceporacin®), cephaprin (Cefadyl®) and cephradine (Velosef®). In general, they are effective against *E. coli, Proteus, Klebsiella, Hemophilus,* and many species of *Staphylococcus* and *Streptococcus.* They are not effective against *Pseudomonas.*

Second-generation drugs include cefaclor (Ceclor®) which can be given orally, cefamandole (Mandol) and cefatoxitin (Metoxin®) which must be administered parenterally. Cefaclor and cefamandole are effective against *E. coli, Klebsiella* and some species of *Staphylococcus* and *Proteus.*

The third generation includes cefoperazone (Cefobid®) and cefotaxime (Claforan®) which must be given parenterally. Their sphere of activity is broadened to include *Citrobacter, Enterobacter, Serratia,* most *Staphylococcus* and *Pseudomonas,* as well as *E. coli, Klebsiella* and *Proteus.*

The development of the later generations of cephalosporins has decreased the need for using the potentially more toxic aminoglycosides.

Aminoglycosides

Aminoglycosides are parenterally administered agents whose development has greatly aided the treatment of serious infections, especially those due to *Pseudomonas, Serratia,* and *Proteus.* They are also effective against *E. coli, Klebsiella, Enterobacter,* and *Staphylococcus* but are seldom effective against streptococci or the anaerobes.

Some members of the aminoglycoside group are gentamicin (Garamycin), amikacin (Amikin®), and tobramycin (Nebcin®).

Allergy to one aminoglycoside usually applies to all.

The potential for toxicity is great, although its likelihood can be diminished by patient selection and careful dosage control. Toxic effects are more frequent in the very young or the very old and with high dosage or prolonged administration. This possibility is increased by sequential or concurrent administration of other aminoglycosides or the simultaneous administration of neuromuscular blocking agents, capreomycin (Capastat®), cisplatin (Platinol®), ethacrynic acid (Edecrin®), furosemide (Lasix), mercaptomerin, vancomycin (Vancocin®), cephalosporins, or polymixin.

Ototoxicity can result in irreversible deafness. Its onset can be detected by daily questioning of the patient about ringing in the ears or decreased hearing. If such symptoms develop, the medication should be stopped. An audiogram made before treatment or during the first two days can be compared with those taken at ten days and six weeks after the beginning of treatment to prevent the mistaken association of future deafness with the aminoglycoside therapy.

Nephrotoxicity should be guarded against by daily urinalyses and serum creatinine determinations. Neuromuscular blockade can be suspected by observing depth of respiration and testing muscle strength.

Aminoglycosides are excreted by the kidneys, but since the rate of clearance differs significantly among individuals, aminoglyoside clearance should be performed before establishing the dosage and timing of administration. Such clearances require good cooperation among the attending physician, the clinical pharmacologist or doctor of pharmacy, and the nursing staff.

The initial dose is the amount usually given to a person with given height, weight and creatinine clearance. The dose is given by intravenous bolus. Blood is then drawn at hourly intervals to determine the occurrence of the highest concentration, called the peak, and the lowest effective concentration, called the trough. From this data, the optimum dosage and the periodicity of administration can be determined.

Aminoglycosides are usually given for ten days. Daily urine cultures will help in the decision regarding the length of the course.

In our experience this regimen has minimized toxicity, although our patient population has not included the very young, the very old or those with renal failure. Nevertheless, the program is expensive and cumbersome, although it can be lifesaving when bacterial resistance precludes the use of other antibiotics. Fortunately, the development of the third-generation cephalosporins has decreased the frequency of need for aminoglycosides.

In summary, preventive or prophylactic treatment of urinary tract infections should emphasize hygienic or dietetic methods but may include the use of urinary acidifiers or small doses of antibacterials.

Suppressive treatment implies toleration of the presence of bacteria but control of their concentration to sub-dangerous levels.

Active treatment seeks to eradicate bacteria by the use of appropriate doses of antibacterials known to be effective for the species present.

As new antibiotics are developed and proven, the more dangerous and less effective drugs should be discarded. It is important that the advantages and disadvantages of each product be remembered and that choice of an antibiotic be based upon its merits rather than on past therapeutic habits.

M.P.

REFERENCES

1. Kevorkian, C.G., Merritt, J.L., and Ilstrup, D.M.: Methanamine mandelate with acidification: An effective urinary antiseptic in patients with neurogenic bladder. *Mayo Clinic Proc* 59:523–529, Aug, 1984.
2. United States Pharmacopeial Convention, Inc.: 1983, Vol. I, Drug Information for the Health Care Provider, Rockville, 1983.

Chapter XIV

PHARMACOLOGICAL MANAGEMENT
OF BLADDER KINETICS

For centuries, physicians and patients have tried to mimic the action of the normal bladder by the use of herbs, potions and drugs. Although there has been considerable progress toward the achievement of this goal, actual results of treatment are often disappointing because of our incomplete understanding of the complex human mechanism, as well as the multi-system effects of the medications.

Today, it is recognized that most bladder dysfunction in the adult results from mechanical obstruction to outflow, local bladder irritation, decreased awareness of bladder fullness or defects of innervation. Although this chapter will emphasize the use of medications[1] to modify such dysfunction, every member of the health team should remember that controlled fluid intake, dietary management, good hygiene, and a time schedule for voiding can often minimize and sometimes obviate the need for drugs in bladder management. Only when behavioral measures fail, or are only partially effective, should medications be considered. With mechanical obstruction, of course, surgical techniques are almost always necessary.

BLADDER IRRITATION

Local bladder irritation often causes painful voiding (dysuria) accompanied by frequency, precipitant voiding or hematuria. Dysuria is common with childhood urinary tract infections as well as with sexual activity, the so-called honeymoon cystitis. Especially in the latter, the urine culture may be negative even though symptoms may strongly suggest infection. In such cases, the causative organism may be an anaerobe or some other of the bacteria for which laboratories do not commonly test. With an anatomically normal bladder, increased fluid intake is often sufficient to flush out the offending organism. If symptoms of pain or tenesmus are prominent, phenazopyridine (Pyridium®) will usually provide analgesia, although the patient should be warned that the urine will become orange and that staining of the underwear will occur. With the neurogenic bladder, such measures are seldom effective. Then the infection should be precisely defined and treated with the appropriate antibacterial. In the absence of infection, stones, foreign bodies, and hormonal changes should be ruled out.

DECREASED AWARENESS OF FULLNESS

Decreased awareness of bladder fullness may be due to brain or spinal cord damage, peripheral nerve changes such as the neuropathies of diabetes and alcoholism, local trauma as that accompanying pelvic surgery, or to the central changes resulting from stroke and old age. In all of these, behavioral training can be of great help, but in the first three conditions drugs are seldom of benefit.

Fortunately, the forgetfulness, somnolence, and short attention span found with advanced age and following some strokes can sometimes be ameliorated by the judicious use of central nervous stimulants such as methylphenadrine (Ritalin®) or caffeine. Such substances must be carefully titrated by an experienced clinician because of the increased sensitivity of the elderly to most medications; however, when skillfully administered, they can be helpful.

DEFECTS IN INNERVATION

The chief uses of pharmaceuticals for bladder control consists of modifying the excessive bladder contractions, stimulating the sluggish bladder contractions or diminishing the sphincter spasticity which accompanies neurologic deficits caused by trauma, ischemia, demyelinization, or congenital defects. Examples of such causative conditions are spinal cord injury, spinal cord tumors or vascular abnormalities, multiple sclerosis, and spina bifida.

Bladder Spasticity

Uncontrolled bladder spasticity results in urinary incontinence which decreases the individual's social acceptability because of wetness and the pervasive odor of urine. Skin irritation and decubitus ulcers may result from such disability. In the past, many were doomed to the use of diapers, urinals, indwelling catheters, or external drainage devices. Even today such arrangements may prove unavoidable, but in many cases, medications make them unnecessary.

Success depends upon careful administration plus cooperation from the patient and the various members of the health team in order to avoid adverse side effects and arrive at optimal dosage. The drugs currently available are anticholinergics with some of the attributes of atropine. Those commonly used are methantheline (Banthine), propantheline (Pro-Banthine) and oxybutynin (Ditropan). Adverse side effects are urinary retention, glaucoma, blurred vision, dry mouth, elevated body temperature due to decreased sweating, constipation, flushing of the skin, drowsiness, nervousness, and decreased sexual ability.

Bladder Atony

Decreased bladder contractility resulting from denervation often responds to the cholinergic drug bethanecol (Urecholine®, Duvoid) provided that significant muscle atrophy or replacement of muscle with fibrous connective tissue have not occurred. It is important not to stimulate bladder contractions in the presence of outlet obstruction because of the dangers of elevated intravesical pressure and reflux. For this reason, some clinicians insist on the simultaneous administration of phenoxybenzamine (Dibenzyline) which inhibits contractility of the lower part of the bladder fundus, internal sphincter, and proximal urethra.

Side effects of oral bethanecol include slow pulse, flushed skin, diarrhea, belching, blurred vision and gastric irritation. Asthmatic attacks may be precipitated and peptic ulcers aggravated. Since some of these side effects are serious, it is especially important to begin with a low dose of bethanecol (usually 10 mg twice daily) and increase it slowly until the optimal effect is realized. Periodic measurement of residual urine is imperative so that complete bladder emptying will be assured.

Functional Outlet Obstruction

Dyssynergia is the term used to describe incoordinated activity of the bladder and its sphincters. Strictly speaking, this term can be used to describe the failure of the bladder to contract when the sphincters relax, but ordinarily it is applied to the opposite situation, the inability of the internal or external sphincter to relax during the voiding contraction of the detrusor. Since active closure of the internal sphincter is accomplished by alpha-adrenergic stimulation, the alpha-adrenergic blocking drug, phenoxybenzamine (Dibenzyline) is used to counteract such stimulation and to permit the internal sphincter to open.

The most common side effect of phenoxybenzamine is orthostatic hypotension. This can usually be avoided by starting treatment with small doses, 5 mg twice daily and increasing the amount by 5-mg increments every four to seven days until the desired effect is achieved. Alcohol should be avoided because it tends to dilate the peripheral circulation increasing the possibility of hypotension.. Other side effects of phenoxybenzamine may be rapid pulse, stuffy nose, dry mouth, diarrhea, drowsiness and the inability to ejaculate.

Dyssynergia may also be the result of spasticity of the skeletal musculature comprising the external sphincter. The muscle relaxants most frequently used are diazepam (Valium), baclofen (Lioresal) or dantrolene (Dantrium).

Diazepam (Valium) is a central nervous system depressant which also has a locally inhibiting effect upon the contractility of skeletal muscle. The exact mechanism is unknown, although it is thought by some to be anticholinergic.

The most troublesome adverse effects of diazepam are psychological and physical dependence, which may be considerable. *Abrupt withdrawal can result in seizures.* Mental depression and confusion may develop and are often exaggerated by alcohol intake or the use of other central nervous system depressants. Headaches, constipation, and a feeling of tiredness or weakness are not uncommon.

The specific site of action of baclofen (Lioresal) is unknown. It probably acts mainly on the spinal cord centers, although it seems to have varying effects upon the higher centers, also.

There is a wide variety of adverse side effects, ranging from bloody or dark urine, chest pain, hallucinations, mental depression, blurred vision, dizziness, diarrhea and muscle weakness to drowsiness. All symptoms should be reported to the physician for possible dosage modification. *As with diazepam, baclofen should not be abruptly discontinued since seizures may result.*

Dantrolene (Dantrium) acts directly upon skeletal muscle, but it also affects the transmission of nerve impulses and acts as a central nervous system depressant. These diverse actions as well as the potential for liver toxicity require that dantrolene be used only with close supervision. The risk for hepatitis appears to be greatest in patients over age 35, especially females who are taking estrogens, and in any patient taking more than 800 mg of dantrolene daily. Hepatitis is most likely to occur between the third and twelfth months of usage.

Side effects indicative of serious consequences are tarry stools, jaundice, bloody or dark urine, severe constipation, mental depression or confusion, phlebitis with swelling of feet or legs, and skin rash. Less serious are mild diarrhea, drowsiness or muscle weakness.

Many of the side effects can be avoided by starting treatment with low doses and increasing the amounts by small increments. Patients should be warned that the achievement of optimal benefits may be slow because of the need for such gradual increases.

In summary, medications are helpful in the management of bladder dysfunction due to localized bladder irritation, decreased awareness of bladder fullness, functional outlet obstruction, and deficits of innervation.

However, medications should not be used until it is apparent that other methods of control have failed. Every drug has side effects which usually can be minimized by careful control of dosage and elimination of concurrent medicines which alter its effectiveness. Awareness of the modes of action of bladder-modifying drugs will be of benefit to the prescriber, the patient, and the supportive health personnel.

M.P.

REFERENCES

1. United States Pharmacopeial Convention, Inc.: USP Dispensing Information, Vol. I Drug Information for the Health Care Provider, Vol. II Advice for the Patient. Rockville, 1983.

Chapter XV

THE ROLE OF NEUROACTIVE DRUGS

During the lifetime of the patient afflicted with a poorly functioning bladder, a variety of medications will be prescribed which intentionally or otherwise mimic the effects of the intact nervous system upon bladder, sphincters, and proximal urethra.

TREATMENT OF NEUROGENIC BLADDER

Five categories of drugs are used to control lower urinary tract function:[1,2]

Cholinergic: increasing the contraction of smooth muscle of bladder and trigone and, sometimes, the somatic muscle of the external sphincter (example: Urecholine).

Anticholinergic: diminishing the contraction of the muscles mentioned above (example: Pro-Banthine).

Alpha adrenergic: contracting internal sphincter and urethra (example: Tofranil®).

Alpha-adrenergic blockers: inhibiting the contraction of internal sphincter and urethra (example: Dibenzylene).

Beta adrenergic: relaxing internal sphincter and urethra and to some extent, the distal detrusor (example: Dibenzylene).

The sixth category is not employed specifically for micturition control but may affect the lower tract through its side effects:

Beta-adrenergic blockers: inhibiting the relaxation of internal sphincter and urethra and, to a lesser degree, the distal detrusor.

NEUROACTIVE DRUGS USED FOR OTHER CONDITIONS

The difficulty of pharmacologic bladder management is multiplied by the interference of many other neuroactive drugs used for common ailments such as allergies, nasal stuffiness, cold symptoms, asthma, diarrhea, constipation, excessive sweating, fever, autonomic dysreflexia, nausea and vomiting, somatic spasticity, anxiety, depression and pain. Such drugs are often prescribed by more than one physician or purchased over the counter.

A drug which duplicates the effect of another is said to be additive, one

229

which negates an activity, antagonistic. If the pitfalls of pharmacological bladder control are to be minimized, it is important that patient and physician be aware of all medications being used and be familiar with their spheres of action.

An example of a common dilemma is the treatment of an incomplete quadriplegic man with a hyporeflexic bladder drained by an external catheter and stimulated by Urecholine. His nasal stuffiness is treated with Ornade®, an alpha-adrenergic and anti-cholinergic drug which, while diminishing nasal congestion, incidentally decreases bladder contractions and may increase sphincter contractility. As a result, urinary retention and bladder over-distension occur to the perplexity of the patient or the health professional who is unaware that two antagonistic drugs are being used.

A somewhat different problem can arise with additive drugs. Consider the woman with hay fever who is also suffering from incontinence due to a hyperreflexic bladder. She is given Pro-Banthine which appears to control the incontinence; however, when hay fever season ends and an antihistamine bought without prescription is discontinued, the incontinence reappears.

Another example is the elderly man with a slightly hypertrophied prostate who develops diarrhea. His physician prescribes Donnatol®. Its anticholinergic effect diminishes bladder contractility just enough so that it cannot force the urine past the obstruction. Urinary retention results.

Because so many medications have neuroactive side effects, it is important that a complete list of drugs being used by a patient be provided to the physician when changes in medication are planned and that the possible interactions of the drugs be considered. Even with great care, conflict may exist because of the different responses of individual patients to various medications.

Table XV–I was designed to aid in identifying drugs which might cancel out the effect of medications used for the pharmacological control of bladder and sphincter function. Although the drugs named are not all-inclusive, the groups listed are sufficient to arouse suspicion of antagonistic action when the desired effect of a program is not achieved.

M.P.

TABLE XV-I
NEUROACTIVE DRUGS AFFECTING THE LOWER URINARY TRACT

Bladder Medication	Desired Effects	Side Effects	Antagonistic Drugs
Cholinergic 　Bethanecol 　　Urecholine® 　　Duvoid®	Increased bladder contractility	Bladder-sphincter dyssynergia Diarrhea Asthma Bradycardia	Anti-allergy 　All antihistamines 　　Benadryl® 　　Phenergan® 　　Ornade® 　　Dimetapp® Sedatives, tranquilizers 　Dalmane® 　Donnatal® 　Elavil® 　Librium® 　Thorazine® 　Valium® Anti-Nausea 　Dramamine® 　Tigan® 　Vistaril® Analgesics 　Darvon® 　Narcotics 　Talwin® Muscle relaxants 　Dantrium® 　Lioresal® 　Valium® Anti-diarrhea 　Banthine® 　Donnatal® 　Pro-Banthine® Anti-Sweating 　Atropine 　Banthine® 　Inversine® Sphincter stimulants 　Ornade® 　Tofranil® Anti-autonomic dysreflexics 　Inversine® 　Ismelin®
Anticholinergic 　Flavoxate 　　Urispas® 　Methantheline 　　Banthine® 　Oxybutynin 　　Ditropan	Decreased bladder contractility	Dry mouth Blurred vision Decreased sweating Headache Constipation	Bladder stimulants 　Duvoid® 　Urecholine® Anti-ileus 　Carbachol® 　Neostigmine® 　Urecholine®

TABLE XV-I (Continued)
NEUROACTIVE DRUGS AFFECTING THE LOWER URINARY TRACT

Bladder Medication	*Desired Effects*	*Side Effects*	*Antagonistic Drugs*
Anticholinergic (*Cont.*) Probantheline Pro-Banthine®			
Alpha-adrenergic Imipramine Tofranil® Pseudoephedrine Sudafed® Ephedrine Ornade®	Increased sphincter tonicity	Nervousness Insomnia Hypertension Autonomic dysreflexia Tachycardia	Anti-autonomic dysreflexia Dibenzyline® Inversine® Ismelin® Serpasil® Sedatives, tranquilizers Elavil® Tofranil® Triavil® Anti-diarrhea Donnatal® Anti-nausea Compazine® Phenergan® Stelazine®
Alpha-adrenergic blocker Phenoxybenzamine Dibenzyline®	Decreased sphincter spasticity	Nasal stuffiness Orthostatic hypotension	Anti-asthmatic Ephedrine Slo-phyllin Gyrotabs® Anti-cold symptoms Actifed® Dimetapp® Ornade® Sudafed® Sinutab® Sedatives, tranquilizers Elavil® Tofranil® Triavil® Anti-Orthostatic Hypotension Ephedrine Propadrine® Sodium Chloride
Beta-adrenergic blocker Phenoxybenzamine Dibenzyline®	Relaxation internal sphincter and proximal urethra	Nasal stuffiness Orthostatic hypo- tension	Anti-dysreflexia Inversine® Ismelin®
Beta-adrenergic blocker Not used to treat urinary problems	Decreased sphincter relaxation		Cardiovascular medications Propranolol

REFERENCES

1. Halstead, L.S., and Claus-Walker, J.: *Neuroactive Drugs of Choice in Spinal Cord Injury.* Houston, The Institute for Rehabilitation and Research, 1980.
2. Goodman, L.S., and Gilman, A.: *The Pharmacologic Basis of Therapeutics.* New York, Macmillan, 1975.

Chapter XVI

MONITORING URINARY TRACT FUNCTION

requent reassessment of the status of the urinary tract is important because deterioration often begins without obvious symptoms.

Patients, families, attendants and hospital or nursing home staff must be made aware of the different ways of monitoring the system and should know the reasons for each procedure. Some tests are simple, some complex, but all help to guarantee good health.

URINARY pH

Testing the urinary pH is easy. Each day a piece of pH paper is moistened with freshly voided urine and after a few seconds the paper is compared with a color-coded chart on its package.

The term pH refers to the concentration of hydrogen ions in a solution, but, for our purpose, it can be used to indicate the degree of acidity or alkalinity of the urine. Often, patients understand more easily if they are reminded that vinegar is acid and baking soda is alkaline.

Healthy persons usually produce acid urine with a pH between 5.0 and 6.5. Seven is the dividing line between acid and alkaline and is called neutral.

Most bacteria do not multiply easily in an acid urine. Moreover, many of the chemicals which form stones stay in solution in an acid urine but precipitate as crystals in an alkaline urine. Therefore, acid urine discourages infections and makes stone formation less likely.

The two most frequent causes of alkaline urine are immoderate consumption of alkaline-ash foods and an infection with urea splitting bacteria. A list of alkaline-and acid-ash foods is in the Appendix. It is not necessary to eliminate alkaline-ash foods completely from the diet, but one should learn to use them with moderation so that the quantities consumed will not be sufficient to change the urine pH from acid to alkaline. If at any time the urine pH shifts from acid to alkaline, the person should review his diet to see if he has eaten or drunk an excess of alkaline-ash foods.

If the pH remains above 7.0 for a day or two and no dietary cause can be found, a urine culture should be made, because the second most common cause of alkaline urine is infection with urea splitting bacteria. These are bacteria which digest urea molecules to produce ammonia and bicarbonate. The most common urea splitters are *Pseudomonas, Proteus* and *Klebsiella.*

Everyone involved in urinary tract care should remember that it is possible to have an infection even if the urine is acid, since not all bacteria split urea.

Patients who have had bladder or kidney stones should be especially careful to keep the urine acid so as to keep crystals from precipitating.

RESIDUAL URINE MEASUREMENT

Residual urine is the amount of urine remaining in a bladder after voiding or in a conduit after expulsion of the urine by peristalsis.

A small post-voiding residual is important to avoid stagnation of urine with growth of bacteria. In the bladder, a residual of less than 50 ml to 100 ml is desirable. An ileal conduit should not have more than 10 ml residual.

If reflux occurs, an infected residuum can cause pyelonephritis.

Measurement of residual urine is made immediately after voiding by an appliance-free person or one using an external collecting device. A catheter is inserted, using sterile technique, and the remaining urine is removed from the bladder by gentle aspiration and measured. The time which has passed since voiding is noted. Since urine is ordinarily excreted at a rate no greater than one to two ml per minute, the true residual can be estimated if one knows the time lapse since voiding.

In an ileal or colonic conduit, the loop measurement is similarly estimated by obtaining the specimen with the sterile double lumen catheter technique.[1] Ten ml residual is the upper limit of normal for an ileal conduit; 20 ml is often quoted for a colonic conduit.

URINALYSIS

Urinalysis should be performed using freshly voided urine, not that which has been taken from a leg bag or ostomy bag, where bacterial growth can change the composition of the urine.

Urinalysis, as well as pH determination, has been greatly simplified by the use of laboratory "sticks" which are dipped into the urine and compared with color charts which indicate the presence of sugar, protein, ketones, blood and bilirubin as well as the pH.

A drop of centrifuged urine is then examined under the microscope to determine the presence of red cells, white cells, casts, crystals, or bacteria. Although all positive findings should be considered seriously, it is usually wise to repeat an abnormal urinalysis to see if the findings are the result of either transient conditions or contamination.

For example, the presence of bacteria is often due to storing the urine in an unsterile container or to delay in processing the specimen. Sugar may be present because of recent excessive intake of sweets, and mild proteinuria may be the result of contamination of the urine by a drop of urethral or vaginal secretion.

URINE CULTURE

Urine is cultured to see if bacteria are growing in the bladder or the kidneys. Consequently, great care must be taken to prevent false results due to contamination of the urine by bacteria in the environment. Methods of obtaining urine for culture are detailed in Chapter XII. After the urine is collected in a sterile receptacle, it is necessary to refrigerate it immediately and to take it to the laboratory within an hour. Since bacteria double in number every 20 to 30 minutes at room temperature, a specimen which remains on a desk or countertop for a long time will contain many more bacteria than were present in the urine at the time it was collected.

The reliability of a urine culture depends considerably upon the manner in which the urine is obtained and the way it is treated before it reaches the laboratory technologist.

ANTIBODY-COATED BACTERIA DETERMINATION (ACB)

In laboratories where it is available, the Antibody-Coated Bacterial Determination test[2] is helpful in interpreting culture results. When the test was first devised it was thought that bacteria which were coated with antibody came only from the kidney. Now, it is believed that antibody production is stimulated by bacterial invasion of any tissue; hence, antibody-coated bacteria may come from the kidney, ureter, bladder wall or prostate.[3] The importance of the test appears to be not for anatomic location of infection in the genitourinary tract as much as for indicating if the bacteria have invaded tissue.[4] Such information can change treatment, since invasive infections often require more vigorous and prolonged treatment than superficial ones.

The Antibody-Coated Bacteria test is not reliable in children because of their immature immunological systems.

URINE LACTIC DEHYDROGENASE DETERMINATION (ULD)

Lactic dehydrogenase is an enzyme which is increased when tissue is damaged by microbial, chemical, mechanical or other means. The total enzyme is made up of five isoenzymes. Normal people may have very small amounts of lactic dehydrogenase in the urine, usually isoenzymes one and two.

A research report[5] suggests that elevated total urinary lactic dehydrogenase with proportionately increased isoenzymes one and two can be detected when there has been urethral or bladder damage, while the isoenzymes four and five are elevated in the presence of kidney pathology. If these hypotheses prove to be correct, an inexpensive and non-invasive method for localizing urinary tract involvement will be available.

ANTIBIOTIC SENSITIVITIES

If the urine culture is positive, antibiotic sensitivity determinations should be ordered to help the doctor select the medication most likely to cure the infection. Each species of bacteria growing in a culture is exposed to measured quantities of several antibiotics. If an antibiotic prevents growth or kills the organism, it is recorded as sensitive. If not, it is called resistant.

It is important to keep records of the species of organisms found in every culture, as well as the antibiotics which are effective. Then, if a patient develops an infection needing immediate treatment, the record of the organisms found in the past, as well as the medications which have proved helpful, make it easier to choose an appropriate antibiotic while awaiting the return of the current culture and sensitivity results.

URODYNAMIC STUDIES

Urodynamic studies graphically portray the mechanical work performed by the lower urinary tract during micturition. Commonly utilized procedures are cystometry, the urethral pressure profile and fluoroscopy or videotaping of the bladder and urethra during voiding.

Cystometry

Cystometry is the measurement of the capacity and contractility of the bladder. Sterile water, sterile normal saline or a gas such as carbon dioxide or air is permitted to flow at a predetermined rate through a catheter into the bladder. A pressure transducer connected to a recorder documents change of intravesical pressure in a tracing which is called a cystometrogram (CMG).

The bladder contraction which occurs when the volume of liquid or gas is large enough to trigger voiding is called a voiding contraction, detrusor contraction, detrusor reflex, or micturition reflex. Artifacts from increases of pressure due to coughing or patient movement are labeled as they occur. The term "bladder capacity" is used to indicate the volume at which the voiding contraction occurs or, in its absence, the volume at which discomfort is present.

The patient's sensation is recorded on the tracing by the technician and includes first sensation of fullness (FSF), final feeling of fullness (FFF), urge to void, and pain. Abnormal sensations such as chills, sweating or headache are also noted.

When gas or fluid is introduced into the normal bladder, there is an abrupt but small rise in pressure which is called the resting pressure (Fig. XVI-1). Since, within limits, the bladder accommodates to increasing volumes without an increased intravesical pressure, there is a prolonged flat area called the tonus limb. When the volume is great enough to provoke the voiding contraction, the pressure increases with a varying degree of abruptness. The detrusor contraction is sustained until voiding occurs or until the subject is able to inhibit it voluntarily.

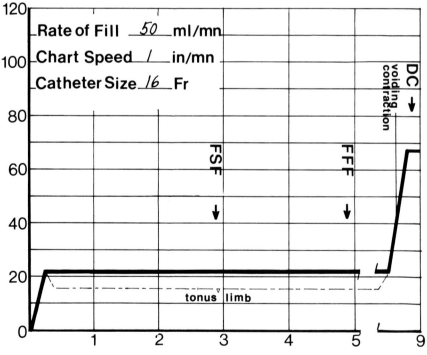

Figure XVI-1. Cystometrogram. Normal bladder.

Usually, an adult is aware of the first sensation of filling at about 150 ml and the final feeling of fullness at about 250 ml. The urge to void generally occurs at about 400 ml and is accompanied by a detrusor contraction of 40 mm or more. Forty-six percent of normal females and 5 percent of normal males do not develop detrusor contractions during cystometry.[6]

Deviations from the normal cystometric tracing are usually due to changes in innervation, although they may result from local conditions in the bladder.

Although the concept is overly simplistic, pathologic changes in the innervation of the bladder are often described as occuring in the "upper motor neurone" or the "lower motor neurone."

Hyperreflexic Bladder (Upper Motor Neurone Lesion)

When the site of neurologic disruption is cephalad to the micturition center in the spinal cord, there is said to be an upper motor neurone lesion. The pathology may be either in the sensory or motor fibers going to micturition centers in the brain stem or brain or in cell bodies within those micturition centers themselves. With an upper motor neurone lesion, there is a reduction or loss of the modifying effects, chiefly inhibitory, of the higher centers upon the function of the micturition reflex (Fig. XVI-2).

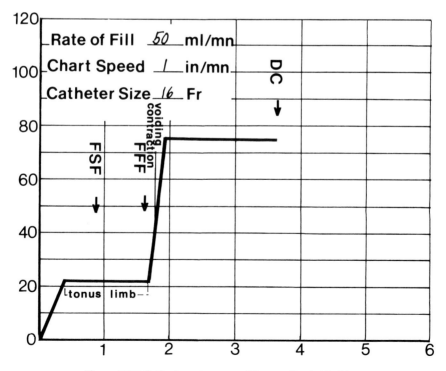

Figure XVI-2. Cystometrogram. Hyperreflexic bladder.

With the lessening of central inhibition, the bladder contracts at a smaller than normal volume of fluid or gas. The contraction occurs abruptly and may be of high amplitude. There may be uninhibited or incoordinated contractions instead of a single sustained contraction. Sensation is absent, decreased, or abnormal. If the lesion is higher than T6, there may be symptoms of autonomic dysreflexia such as chills, sweating, headache, or rise of blood pressure.

Hyporeflexic Bladder (Lower Motor Neurone Lesion)

When the site of neurologic disruption is in or distal to the spinal micturition center, there is said to be a hyporeflexic or lower motor neurone bladder. The pathologic process may be found in the sensory fibers going to the center, in the nerve cells of the center itself or in the motor fibers going to the bladder. In any of these circumstances, the bladder will not contract when filled. However, if the sensory fibers and cell bodies are not involved while the motor fibers are defective, the patient will feel the desire to void but will be unable to do so. The cystometrographic tracing of a hyporeflexic bladder will show a gradually ascending tonus limb with no micturition contraction (Fig. XVI-3).

With both upper or lower motor neurone bladders there may be either complete or incomplete neurologic lesions. If some portions of the reflex arcs between sites of bladder stimulation and bladder contraction remain functional, the lesion is called incomplete. A tracing of a bladder with incomplete innervation will vary depending on the proportion of nerve fibers or cell bodies which are affected.

Serial cystometrograms made every one to two weeks following spinal cord injury are useful in signaling the end of spinal shock. During post-hospital discharge follow-up, the cystometrogram can give clues to unsuspected bladder dysfunction as well as to re-innervation.

In denervating disease such as diabetes, multiple sclerosis, or spinal cord tumors, the cystometrogram may give early warnings of the pathologic processes. Etiology of the incontinence found in aging or after stroke may be clarified by cystometry.

Urethral Pressure Profile

The urethral pressure profile is obtained by drawing a catheter equipped with one or more pressure transducers through the bladder neck and urethra during voiding. The tracing is compared with a normal one to locate functional or mechanical obstruction to outflow.[7]

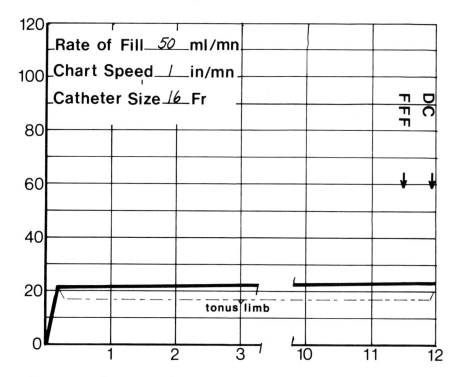

Figure XVI-3. Cystometrogram. Hyporeflexic bladder.

RADIOLOGIC STUDIES

The cystourethrogram (CUG) and the intravenous pyelogram (IVP) are often scheduled during the same x-ray appointment. The cystourethrogram precedes the intravenous pyelogram in order to avoid the problems of interpretation which are introduced if delayed excretion of the dye from the pyelogram outlines a kidney pelvis or ureter during the cystourethrogram simulating vesicoureteral reflux.

Cystourethrogram (CUG)

A cystourethrogram is ordered to determine the presence of bladder stones, changes in bladder morphology and vesicoureteral reflux.

Prior to dye instillation, a scout film (sometimes called plain film) is made to detect the presence of lightly calcified bladder stones which might be overshadowed by the density of the dye (Fig. XVI-4). Radiopaque dye is introduced through a catheter (Fig. XVI-5). When the bladder is filled to capacity, interpretations of trabeculation and saccule formation are more accurate than in the bladder only partially filled with dye (Fig.

XVI-6). Although detection of calculi is important, the major bonus in the cystourethrogram is the visualization of vesicoureteral reflux, the retrograde flow of dye or urine from the bladder toward the kidney (Fig. XVI-7). If the reflux reaches the kidney pelvis it is called complete; if it only goes part way it is called incomplete or partial. If the refluxing ureters and kidney pelvis have become dilated, the condition is called hydronephrosis (Fig. XVI-8).

Intravenous Pyelogram (IVP)

The intravenous pyelogram is also preceded by a scout or plain film to determine kidney size and shape as well as the presence of kidney, ureteral or bladder calculi. Radiopaque dye is injected into the veins of the patient (Fig. XVI-9). Serial films document the time of dye excretion and the morphology of the hollow portions of the kidneys, ureters and bladder. The cup-shaped areas into which the pyramids of the kidney empty should have sharply delineated edges. If these areas, called calyces, appear to be blunt or mis-shapen, tomograms may be made to determine if the change is actual or is an illusion due to the plane in which the calyx lies. The films should include views of the bladder so that its volume can be estimated and the mucosal pattern observed. Vesicoureteral reflux cannot be determined by the intravenous pyelogram. An intravenous pyelogram should not be ordered for patients allergic to iodides.

Since morphologic changes in the kidneys occur slowly, many investigators believe that in the absence of special indications it is not necessary to make an intravenous pyelogram more often than every two years, while a cystourethrogram may be needed more frequently if reflux development is a concern.

RENAL FUNCTION STUDIES

Renal function studies are an important part of the monitoring process because good kidney function is the ultimate goal of urinary tract management.

The parameters of renal function commonly estimated are glomerular filtration rate (GFR), renal plasma flow (RPF) and maximal tubular function (Tm).[8]

The glomerular filtration rate designates the amount of water which the kidneys filter from the blood per minute.

The renal plasma flow denotes the amount of plasma which traverses the kidneys per minute. Estimation of renal plasma flow is generally preferred to renal blood flow, because the variability of the quantity of hemoglobin in the blood has made difficult the establishment of normal values for renal blood flow.

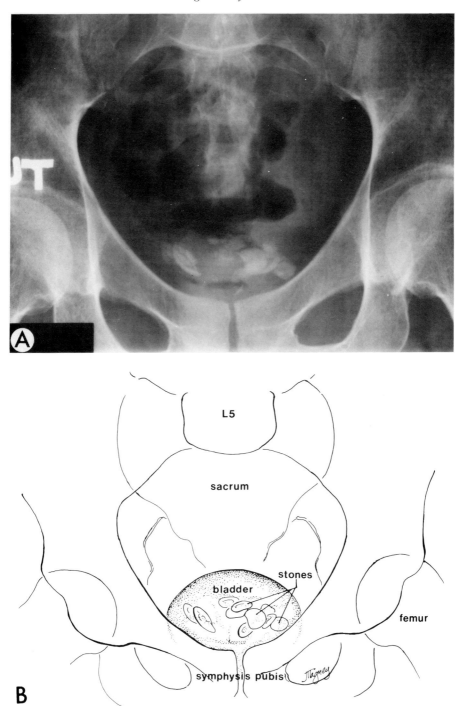

Figure XVI-4 A–B. Cystourethrogram. Scout film showing bladder stones. A. X ray. B. Line drawing.

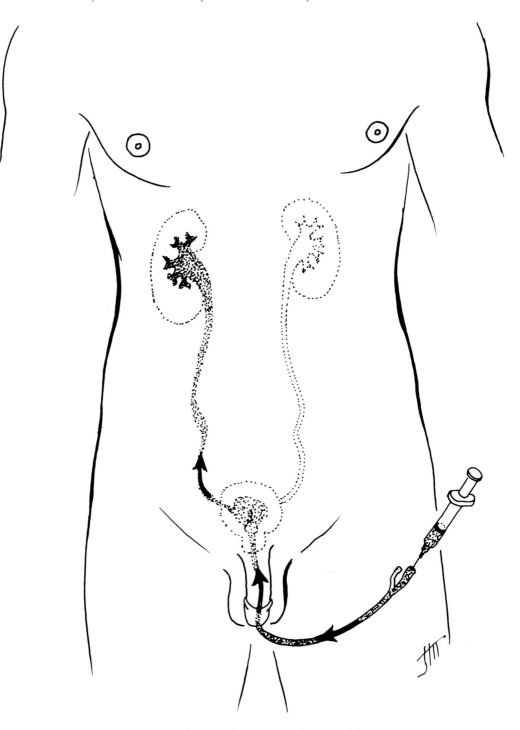

Figure XVI-5. Cystourethrogram. Instillation of dye.

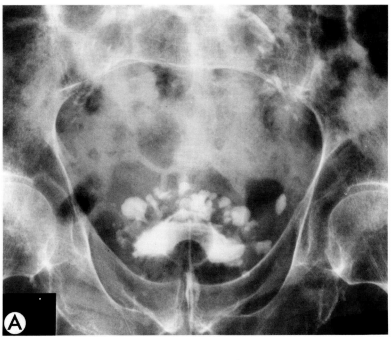

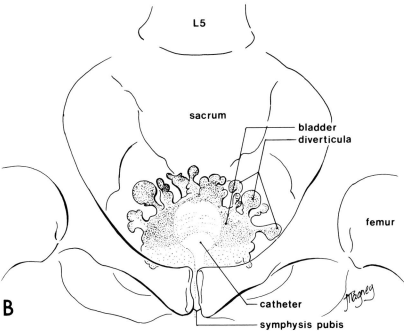

Figure XVI-6 A–B. Cystourethrogram. Trabeculation and sacculation. A. X ray. B. Line drawing.

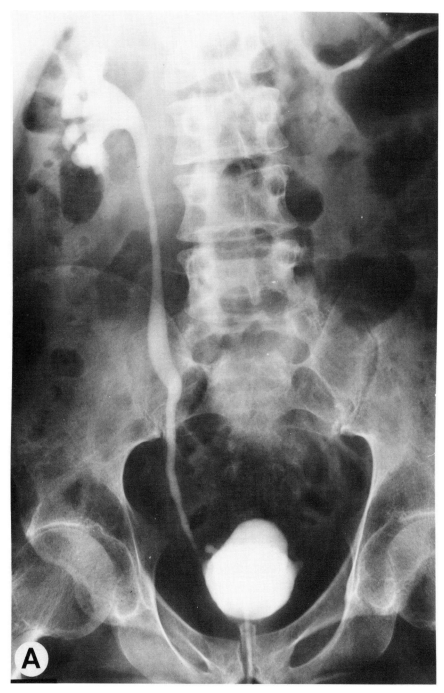

Figure XVI-7 A–B. Cystourethrogram. Complete reflux. A. X ray. (*Opposite Page*) B. Line drawing.

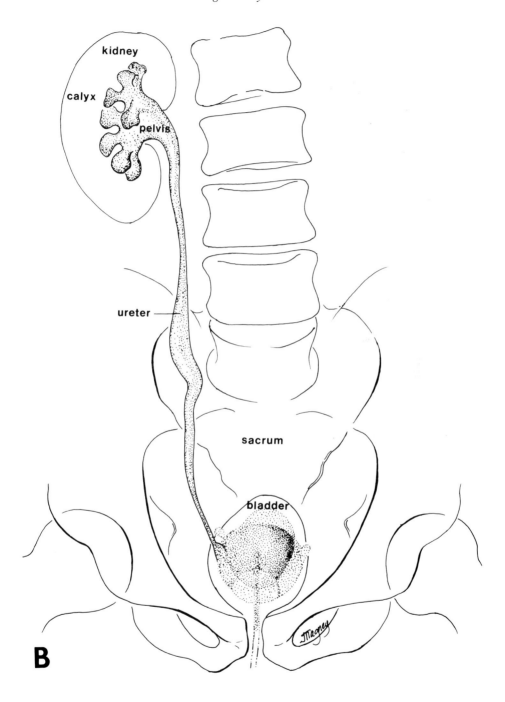

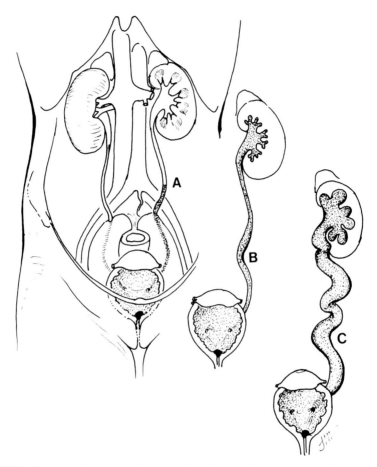

Figure XVI-8. Cystourethrogram. Degrees of reflux. A. Incomplete reflux. B. Complete reflux. C. Hydronephrosis.

Maximal tubular function relates to either absorbtive or excretory capacities. Glucose is resorbed by the tubules and para-aminohippurate (PAH) is excreted. Resorption and excretion are equally affected by most tubular disorders. Since the laboratory determination of para-amino hippurate is simpler than that of glucose, the TmPAH is the test more often used.

In the chronically impaired urinary tract, glomerular filtration rate is likely to deteriorate before tubular function or renal plasma flow.[9] Therefore, the use of a precise indicator of glomerular function is essential.

The inulin clearance fulfills all the physiologic criteria for determining the glomerular filtration rate. Inulin is removed from the blood almost entirely by the glomerulus and is not excreted or resorbed by any other part

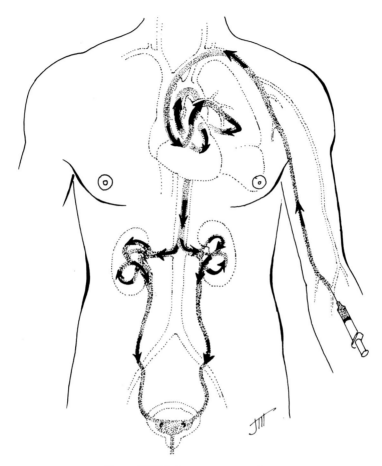

Figure XVI-9. Intravenous pyelogram.

of the nephron. Laboratory determination is simple, and there are no systemic side effects. The inulin clearance has the disadvantage of being time consuming. It is not appropriate for frequent repetitions during episodes of acute pathology because of the need for constant infusion of inulin over a period of an hour to an hour and a half. However, it is a useful and accurate tool in periodic monitoring of glomerular filtration rate.

The 24-hour endogenous creatinine clearance has the advantages of needing only one blood specimen and not requiring intravenous infusion. However, accurate collection of the 24-hour urine specimen is often difficult. Creatinine is excreted by both the glomerulus and the tubule and may also be reabsorbed by the tubule. The unpredictable ratio of tubular secretion and reabsorption (of creatinine) to its glomerular filtration makes creatinine clearance an imprecise method of determining the glomerular filtration rate.

Non-clearance methods of glomerular filtration rate, such as the determination of radioisotopes, are complicated by their unpredictable rate of release from the various body compartments.

Serum creatinine and blood urea nitrogen (BUN) determinations are of use only in the presence of advanced renal deterioration. The blood urea nitrogen is reliable only when the glomerular filtration rate has deteriorated to the fourth standard deviation below the normal mean, and the serum creatinine is reliable only when the glomerular filtration rate has reached the third standard deviation below the normal mean.[9]

Renal plasma flow can be measured simultaneously with glomerular filtration rate by an accompanying infusion of a small concentration of para-aminohippurate.

In an effort to find an easy, safe and economical method for determining glomerular filtration rate and rate of renal plasma flow, many other methods have been evaluated, but, at this writing, none have been without drawbacks.

Since in the chronically impaired patient tubular function does not deteriorate until after the glomerular filtration rate is considerably reduced, the maximal tubular excretory rate (TmPAH) is seldom determined except in the presence of moderate to severely reduced glomerular filtration. The injection of the required amount of paraaminohippurate is often accompanied by a short period of discomfort when the patient feels flushed and warm. Sometimes, headache, abdominal cramps, nausea and occasionally defecation occur. In some patients none of these symptoms develop. After ten to fifteen minutes, the symptoms disappear.

Summary

We recommend that urinary tract function in patients with neurogenic bladders or supravesical diversions be monitored by means of these techniques:

1. Urinary pH determinations
2. Residual urine measurements
3. Urinalysis
4. Urine cultures
5. Urodynamics, emphasizing cystometry
6. Cystourethrograms
7. Intravenous pyelograms
8. Evaluations of kidney function

Educating patients, families, attendants, and health professionals regarding the reasons for the monitoring procedures will result in greater patient compliance.

M.P.

REFERENCES

1. Newman, E., and Price, M.: *Double Lumen Catheterization of the Ileal Conduit: A Manual for Physicians and Health Personnel.* Dept. Physical Medicine and Rehabilitation, University of Minnesota, Minneapolis, 1974, p. 2.
2. Thomas, V., Shelokov, A., and Farland, M.: Antibody-coated bacteria in the urine and the site of urinary tract infection. *N Eng J Med 290:*588, 1974.
3. Jones, S.R.: Prostatitis as cause of antibody-coated bacteria in urine. *N Eng J Med 291:*365, 1974.
4. Newman, E., Price, M., and Ederer, G.: Urinary tract infection in patients with spinal cord lesions: Antibody-coated bacteria tests as a diagnostic aid. *Arch Phys Med and Rehab 61:*406, 1980.
5. Newman, E., Ibrahim, G., and Price, M.: Urine lactic dehydrogenase—An aid in the management of patients with spinal cord injury. *Int Rehabil Med 6:*170, 1984.
6. Merrill, D., Markland, C., and Price, M.: Air Cystometry. *Arch Phys Med and Rehab 54:*393, 1973.
7. Andersen, J., and Bradley, W.: Electromyographic and gas urethral pressure profile. *Urol 7:*561, 1976.
8. Smith, H.: *Principles of Renal Physiology.* New York, Oxford University Press 1962.
9. Price, M.: The inulin clearance as a screening test of kidney function. *Arch Phys Med and Rehab 55:*522, 1974.
10. Price, M., and Kottke, F.J.: Comparison of glomerular filtration rate, blood urea nitrogen and serum creatinine in patients with chronic urinary tract disease. *Minn Med 63:*781, 1980.

Chapter XVII

COMPLICATIONS OF LONG-TERM
URINARY TRACT CARE

The complications of urinary tract care are numerous, among the most common being infection, stone or calculus formation, residual urine, overdistention, vesicoureteral reflux, autonomic dysreflexia, and cancer of the bladder.

INFECTION

The causes, detection, and treatment of infection are treated at length in Chapters II and XI as well as being referred to in the chapters dealing with the various methods of urinary tract drainage. Consequently, this important entity will not be addressed in this chapter except as it contributes to other complications.

URINARY CALCULI

Urinary calculi often plague patients with neurogenic bladders. With care they can be avoided. The extra effort which prevention entails is amply rewarded by the increased well-being of the patient.

The detrimental effects of stones include urinary tract obstruction, infection, pain and spasticity.

Obstruction occurs at the site of formation when the stone has enlarged enough to block that portion of the urinary tract. If motion or gravity dislodges the stone, it can become wedged in a narrower segment below the site of origin (Fig. XVII-1).

Obstruction results not only in urinary stasis and infection but in a rise of hydrostatic pressure which, if prolonged, causes dilatation of the parts above the obstruction and, eventually, destruction of kidney parenchyma.

Even in the absence of obstruction and stasis, stones are often responsible for infections which defy treatment. Crystals accumulate about aggregations of bacteria or infected material such as pus. As layers are deposited, bacteria adhere and are trapped in the body of the stone to be released if conditions favor stone dissolution (Fig. XVII-2). Similarly, bacteria grow in the rough

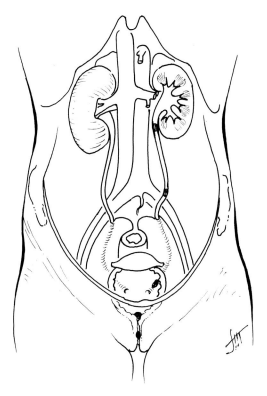

Figure XVII-1. Urinary calculi. Sites of obstruction.

crevices of the outer layer where they are protected from the action of antibiotics to re-seed the urine when treatment stops.

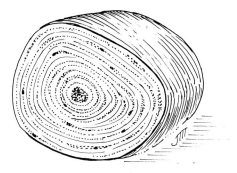

Figure XVII-2. Urinary calculus. Bacterial entrapment.

Patients with good sensation experience exquisite pain when small, sharp stones travel down the ureters or through the urethra. Narcotics are usually required to relieve the pain or to relax the spasticity of smooth muscle about the stones.

The combination of irritation by bladder calculi plus the infections which they perpetuate frequently cause bladder spasms which can be devastating to voiding programs.

In patients with upper motor neurone lesions, somatic spasticity is often severe, particularly in the lower extremities. If stones are not suspected, the etiology of such spasticity can be perplexing and the patient may be futilely subjected to the expense and side effects of muscle-relaxant drugs.

There are many causes for stone formation.[1] Metabolic disorders such as gout or hyperparathyroidism, although uncommon, must be ruled out. The inability to metabolize ascorbic acid without excessive urinary oxylate crystal formation may exist. Immobility encourages the removal of excessive amounts of skeletal calcium which are excreted by the kidneys. Immoderate ingestion of dairy products and alkaline-ash foods may be a factor.

For the most part, stones can be prevented if a dilute urine is maintained, acid urinary pH is sustained and urinary tract infections are avoided.

Normally, urine contains many of the substances found in stones: calcium, magnesium, ammonium, phosphates, carbonates and oxylates. As long as such materials stay in solution, there is no need for concern. When a greater amount of any substance accumulates in the urine than can be kept in solution, the urine is said to be supersaturated and crystalization will occur. Stones cannot be formed in the absence of a supersaturated solution. The way to avoid supersaturation is to keep the urine dilute and to provide an acid pH, since most of the stone-forming chemicals stay in solution more readily if the urine is not alkaline. An additional benefit from dilute urine is the more efficient washout its greater volume provides for the removal of bacteria, crystals and other potential nuclei for stone formation.

Infection encourages calculus formation by supplying bacterial clumps, small blood clots and clusters of white cells which attract crystals. Certain bacteria form urease which splits urea, producing an alkaline urine favoring crystalization.

Urinary stasis within saccules or diverticula provides a haven in which stone formation can commence.

Treatment of existing stones begins with enforcement of the principles just discussed for prevention. Sometimes these measures are enough to dissolve small stones. Usually, however, more heroic approaches are necessary.

During the past few years, there has been considerable innovative effort toward the treatment of urinary stones in an attempt to decrease or eliminate invasive measures with their attendant surgical risks. Since any discussion of the specifics of treatment will quickly become obsolete as new developments occur, only the broad aspects will be considered here.

In the past, bladder stones have conventionally been removed by inserting a cystoscope, grasping the stones with an instrument, crushing them, and flushing out the fragments with a copious flow of sterile water or saline. Stones in the lower third of the ureter were similarly removed. Calculi higher in the ureter or in the kidney, as well as bladder stones which were too large to be crushed, were removed by incision and extraction, often with the accompaniment of considerable morbidity.

Such methods are still the mainstay of stone removal, but other means are emerging which, with the improvements that come with time and experience, should replace many of the surgical approaches and their discomforts and dangers.

Acetohydroxamic acid[2, 3] has recently been released for clinical use as an oral medication for dissolving stones. Undoubtedly, continued research will improve this product and develop other drugs for this purpose.

Irrigation of the kidney in order to dissolve stones, once abandoned because of the dangers of overwhelming infection, has now been resumed with improvements of methodology.

The use of ultrasound to break up calculi by percutaneous or invasive lithotripsy presents another revolutionary development in the treatment of urinary stones.

Such methods, together with the use of new generations of antibiotics for controlling infections, are bound to transform the treatment of urinary stones. Together, with problem recognition and application of the principles of prophylaxis, the health and well-being of persons with neurogenic bladders should increase immeasurably.

RESIDUAL URINE

Residual urine is the amount of urine remaining in the bladder at the end of micturition. It is measured by inserting a catheter and aspirating the bladder contents. The normal bladder empties completely leaving no residual, but since one to two ml of urine are excreted each minute, five to ten ml will be aspirated, depending upon the length of time required for catheterization.

To gain an accurate estimate of the residual, it is essential to know the exact time lapse between cessation of voiding and the end of urine aspiration. The patient or attendant must record both times. (See p 235)

A journal should be kept of the estimated residuals, so that changes of the emptying pattern will be recognized. A consistent increase in the amount of residual suggests either obstruction to outflow or deterioration of neurologic function, indicating the need for a more effective method of drainage or the use of pharmacologic, mechanical, or surgical methods for altering bladder function.

For example, let us consider an appliance-free person who for some time has voided efficiently after suprapubic tapping but who has developed an increasingly large residual. The simple addition of suprapubic pressure may correct the situation, but if it fails, formal investigation of bladder function is mandatory. The cystometrogram may show an elevated threshold for the micturition reflex, in which case cholinergic drugs could be used to increase detrusor contraction. On the other hand, if the urethral pressure profile suggests sphincter fibrosis or spasticity, a sphincterotomy may be indicated. Still another option is the use of intermittent catheterization.

Another benefit from residual urine measurement may be the discovery that asymptomatic overdistention exists. Many patients believe that they are actively urinating when in actuality they are experiencing overflow voiding, i.e. the urine is expelled only when the intravesical pressure exceeds the urethral opening pressure; the flow stops when the bladder pressure drops below that level. Under these conditions, infection almost always exists since washout is impossible.

Conversely, decrease of residual urine may herald improvement of bladder function, although one should be cautioned that the irritating effect of infection can stimulate bladder contractions temporarily.

Still another bonus from monitoring the amount of residual urine is the provision of a guide for regulating fluid intake and frequency of bladder emptying.[4,5]

Finally, knowing the amount of urinary residual helps to determine the need for long-term bacterial suppression, as discussed in Chapter XIII. The larger the residual, the more likely are recurrences of infection and the dangers of bacterial invasion of tissue or bloodstream with subsequent fibrosis, scarring, reflux and stone formation, or, in the case of bloodstream invasion, morbidity or death.

Clinicians sometimes object to measuring residual urine because of the danger of introducing bacteria into the bladder via the catheter. We have not been impressed with this danger providing that unfailing attention is directed toward fastidious cleansing of the meatal and perineal areas, as well as a determined effort to avoid contamination of the sterile catheter. In cases particularly at risk, we have followed the catheterization with twenty-four-hour oral administration of macro-crystaline nitrofurantoin, a drug which is eliminated solely by the kidneys and which is usually effective against *E. coli*. If there is a sensitivity to nitrofurantoin, we have used trimethroprim-sulfonamide preparations. Choice of prophylactic drugs will undoubtedly vary as newer medications are developed.

In summary, measurement of residual urine is important as an indication of the beginning, decrease or improvement of bladder efficiency. Such knowledge can be used to modify treatment of bladder dysfunction as well as to control infection and its sequellae. Residual measurement is safe if performed meticulously, although in some cases concurrent antibiotic administration is beneficial.

OVERDISTENTION

Overdistention occurs when the bladder is filled to greater-than-normal capacity, either from too great an inflow of urine or from a diminished volume of urinary outflow.

As the volume increases beyond capacity, the intravesical hydrostatic pressure rises until minute tears in the lining epithelium develop, rupturing capillaries, venules or arterioles with consequent microscopic or gross hematuria. If bacteria are present, they gain access to the wall of the bladder, setting up infection. Even in the absence of bacteria, the penetrating urine causes a chemical irritation. Scarring follows the inflammation and replaces muscle fibres. If overdistention persists, the increased pressure stretches the fibrous connective tissue, thinning the wall, permitting diverticulum formation and creating incompetence of the ureteral orifices, later leading to reflux.

An acute episode of distention in a functioning bladder can disable the detrusor muscle for periods ranging from an hour to several weeks. Such a situation is particularly disastrous in a bladder recovering from spinal shock, as it may delay rehabilitation and even cause the novice to abandon efforts aimed at encouraging normal function.

Overdistention can be avoided by applying the general principles of prevention to any method of bladder drainage which has been selected.

Each patient must be taught to maintain fluid intake by uniform volumes evenly spaced throughout the day. Such a regimen will provide steady bladder washout and lessen the danger of distention from episodes of increased urine flow accompanying large amounts of fluid intake. For instance, if 2000 ml is the desired daily intake, four portions of 400 ml during the day and one of 400 ml during the night will provide more even urine production than 1000 ml in the morning and 1000 ml in the evening.

An inconsistent rate of urine production can also result from variations in mealtime or recreational food and drink. High sodium foods, such as potato chips or salted peanuts, cause retention of fluid in the tissues with delayed release into the bloodstream and subsequent uneven urine excretion causing unexpected bladder filling. Drinking larger than usual amounts of tea, coffee, or other caffeinated beverages will cause diuresis for which the patient has not provided when planning the schedule for bladder emptying.

Alcoholic beverages also disrupt voiding regimens by several mechanisms. To begin with, alcohol affects the central nervous system by inhibiting the antidiuretic hormone. The purpose of antidiuretic hormone is to prevent the kidney tubules from secreting too much water. Alcohol inhibits this "braking" influence, promoting excretion of large amounts of dilute urine. In addition, the total volume consumed is often large, especially with beverages such as beer and ale. A person drinking a six pack of beer not only sustains the antidiuretic effect equivalent to six "shots" of whiskey but increases his fluid intake by more than two quarts.

Alcohol also has been shown to have other central effects, for example, inhibiting the bladder[6] by raising its threshold to the stimulus of filling. Furthermore, the sedative effect of alcohol may make the drinker less aware of the signs of bladder distention, contributing to neglect of bladder emptying.

Edema is another factor affecting the rate of urine formation, especially if tissue fluid is permitted to pool in dependent lower extremities. With the improved venous and lymphatic return which occurs when the legs are elevated at bedtime, the so-called night diuresis occurs.

Changes in emotional state can cause variations in the rate of urine secretion as well as the efficiency of bladder contractility by affecting the activity of the autonomic nervous system.

The role of obstruction in the development of overdistention must be remembered. Because of its omnipresence as a cause of vesicoureteral reflux, it will be discussed in detail in the next segment of this chapter.

VESICOURETERAL REFLUX

Vesicoureteral reflux is the backward flow of urine from the bladder toward the kidneys (Fig. XVI-6). It is called *incomplete reflux* if the urine goes only part way up the ureter and *complete* if the urine reaches the kidney, itself. If the kidney and ureter become dilated, the term hydronephrosis is used. Some workers classify reflux by grades: Grade I denotes incomplete reflux; Grade II indicates complete reflux with no dilatation; Grade III, complete reflux with mild dilatation; and Grade IV, complete reflux with gross hydroureter and hydronephrosis.

Reflux is dangerous because it permits bacterial ascent from the bladder through the ureters to the kidneys, where infection can not only destroy the functional units but can cause fibrosis of the interstitium which in turn destroys more nephrons as the scar tissue contracts applying pressure to the units and their vascular supply.

As the bacteria are carried past the trigone and through the ureters, some species release toxins which paralyze the smooth muscle of the vesicoureteral valve and the ureter. As a result, the valve becomes less competent, and peristaltic action of the ureters and pelvis is impaired, permitting elevated hydrostatic pressure throughout the upper tracts with stagnation of urine, conducive both to infection and stone formation.

The immediate cause of reflux is incompetency of the valve formed by smooth muscle at the trigonal juncture of the ureter and the bladder (see Chap. I). When the normal bladder is full or when it contracts to produce voiding, the lower end of the ureter is closed to prevent urine from being forced into the ureter. The vesico-ureteral junction loses its competence by several means.

Congenital defects can result in abnormal function or placement of the muscle fibres which make up the functional valve (see Chap. I). In other instances the distal ureter fails to traverse the bladder wall in the diagonal path which helps to assure ureteral closure as detrusor muscle strands tighten in response to increased tension. More often, reflux is the product of infection, obstruction to outflow causing overdistention, or a combination of the two.

Acute infection produces edema and engorgement of the bladder muscosa, altering the smooth surface necessary for tight closure of the ureteral orifices. Bacterial toxins may also lessen the contractile power of the smooth muscle fibres which tighten about the openings. Periodically, the irritating effect of infection can also create or increase bladder spasticity so that the augmented voiding contraction greatly increases intravesical pressure just prior to urine expulsion, further stressing the valve.

With recurrent or chronic infection, detrusor and ureteral muscle fibres may be replaced by fibrous connective tissue which alters the effectiveness of valve closure. Early, the bladder wall can hypertrophy providing contractions sufficient to empty the partially fibrosed bladder, but eventually the bladder becomes a sacculated bag unable to cope with increasing pressures. On the other hand, the fibrous connective tissue may shorten leaving the patient with a thickened, small volume bladder. If the sphincters also constrict preventing outflow, reflux will result.

Obstruction can be either external, anatomical or functional. In the past, elderly, incontinent men were subjected to a constrictive device, called the Cunningham clamp, which was placed about the penis so as to compress the urethra. The instrument not only caused urethral trauma leading to stricture but pressure sores. Fortunately, its use has been practically eliminated.

Today, most external obstruction results from the faulty use of urinary drainage appliances. With external catheters, the bands or tapes provided to secure the sheath to the shaft of the penis may be applied too tightly. Indwelling urethral or suprapubic catheters can be plugged by mucous, blood clots, calcific deposits or other detritus. The bags or containers into which catheters or conduits drain may become so full that the constantly forming urine cannot escape and bladders or conduits become overdistended.

Twisting, kinking or compression of any part of a drainage system will have a similar effect.

Anatomical obstruction has many causes. Urethral strictures often follow urethritis, either venereal or non-venereal, but may be the result of trauma such as urethral compression during difficult childbirth. One of the most frequent causes of bladder outlet obstruction is the benign prostatic hypertrophy developing in men over sixty. With an increasing geriatric population among both able-bodied and disabled people, this form of obstruction will become even more common. Malignant tumors are less numerous, but they too can cause obstruction. Urinary tract stones lodging in the urethra or lying over its internal opening can obstruct the bladder outlet. In the latter case, obstruction may be intermittent, decreasing when the stone falls away from the urethral orifice as the patient shifts position.

Functional obstruction derives from the failure of the internal or external sphincters to relax in coordination with the voiding contraction or from the inability of the detrusor to produce a contraction forceful enough to overcome the opening pressure of the sphincters. In either case, the product is overdistention of the bladder. Intravesical pressure may increase until the sphincters are forced to open and overflow voiding occurs or until the opening pressure of the vesicoureteral junction is exceeded and reflux occurs. Either circumstance may be accompanied by autonomic dysreflexia. Both forms of functional obstruction are usually the result of neurologic dysfunction.

Normal sphincter opening depends upon the ability of the smooth muscle of the internal sphincter and the striated muscle of the external sphincter to relax, permitting urine to escape when the detrusor contracts. Consequently, spasticity of either the internal or external sphincter will prevent urinary outflow. Such spasticity is frequently found in quadriplegia due to spinal cord injury or brain injury or in multiple sclerosis and can be exacerbated by any noxious influence.

Contractile incapacity of muscle fibres and diminution of nervous stimuli both produce a flaccid, impotent bladder wall, as real an obstruction as the inability of a sphincter to open. Fiber weakness can result from disuse or disease. Isolation from nervous stimuli can be central because of brain or spinal cord damage, peripheral from the neuropathies of diabetes, alcoholism or heavy metal exposure, or hormonal due to endogenous or exogenous blockade of cell receptors.

Since prevention of any condition begins with alertness to its likelihood, realization of the potential for development of reflux should sensitize patient and health care providers to the presence of inauspicious circumstances, spurring them on to eradicate such conditions before deterioration takes place.

Congenital defects are the most difficult to prevent, since prophylactic measures must be instituted before the birth of offspring. As knowledge expands, genetic counseling becomes more effective, and protection of the fetus is made more feasible through good nutrition and the avoidance of alcohol, tobacco and other deleterious substances.

Infection prevention is discussed in Chapter XI. To summarize, urinary tract infection can nearly always be avoided by awareness of the sites of bacterial access in each kind of urinary tract drainage plus the application of principles of cleanliness, gentle handling, avoidance of overdistention, and provision of sufficient fluid washout.

The prevention of obstruction to outflow depends upon knowledge of its cause and its pattern of development. Since in many cases obstruction cannot be entirely prevented, monitoring for progression becomes extremely important.

Obstruction due to external causes can be eliminated in part by vigilance regarding the patency of the urethra and all tubes or devices leading from or attached to the bladder or urinary diversion. The patient with a recently disabled bladder may be so overwhelmed by floods of instruction that basics, such as keeping drainage lines straight and unimpinged, are overshadowed. As the years pass, commonplace items tend to be forgotten. One role of the health care provider is to reinforce defective memories.

Preventing anatomical obstruction is a more complex problem. Strictures due to venereal urethritis can be avoided by care in the choice of sexual partners and by prompt treatment of contracted infections. The sources of non-venereal urethral infections are often unidentifiable, but immediate treatment is essential in order to prevent urethral scarring. Many strictures follow urethral trauma, principally due to instrumentation. They can be avoided by keeping catheterization, cystoscopy and passage of urethral sounds to a minimum, lubricating each instrument well and inserting it gently.

Obstruction from tumors or prostatic hypertrophy must be discovered by observation of urine flow characteristics as well as by symptom recognition. In the otherwise non-disabled person, difficulty in passing urine, bladder distention and hematuria will be recognized by discomfort or visual cues. The disabled person, however, may remain unaware of such developments either because of inability to perceive pain or by the masking of urinary flow characteristics by drainage devices. In such cases, observation must be expanded to include palpation of the bladder, deliberate inspection of the urine, periodic rectal examination, and more formal monitoring procedures such as x-ray and pressure studies.

Prevention of functional obstruction requires even more expertise. As a result, great cooperation and adequate communication among physician, nurse, attendants, family, patient and other members of the health team must be promoted.

The flaccid bladder can often be avoided by preventing overdistention. Atrophy of disuse of the bladder wall caused by deprivation of nerve supply can sometimes be prevented through the use of medications which mimic the actions of excitatory neurotransmission or which block the effects of inhibiting transmitters (see Chap. XV).

Spasticity of the bladder sphincters is almost always due to neurologic deficits and, hence, is often not amenable to prophylactic measures, although exacerbation of spasticity can be avoided by eliminating irritating conditions such as infection, pressure sores and psychologic stress.

Treatment of reflux is varied and depends considerably upon the degree of deterioration as well as its cause. It responds less readily to conservative treatment in adults than in children.

Congenital defects of ureteral placement are generally amenable to surgical treatment provided the ureters as well as the bladder wall have not been too greatly damaged by infection or increased pressure. Ureteral reimplantation is usually the treatment of choice, although cystoplasty or ureteroplasty may sometimes be necessary.

Non-congenital reflux, especially in the early stages, will often be alleviated by elimination of infection (See Chap. XI) and correction of obstruction by providing good urinary drainage.

Anatomical obstruction nearly always requires a surgical approach rather than a medical one. Urethral strictures can sometimes be stretched by the use of sounds. Bladder stone removal has been discussed.

Benign prostatic hypertrophy is treated surgically, the technique varying with the degree of enlargement. Treatment of cancer of the prostate depends upon the stage of the cancer and the degree of obstruction. Frequently, a combination of surgery, radiation, hormonal therapy and chemotherapy is used. Intravesical neoplasms are subjected to surgery, radiation or chemotherapy, often in combination.

Treatment of functional obstruction is seldom simple because of the intricacies of physiological control. Intermittent catheterization may fail because of the tendency of the internal sphincter to go into spasm at the touch of the catheter, preventing free passage of the catheter and often inducing autonomic dysreflexia. Indwelling uretheral or suprapubic catheterization is avoided because of the dangers of infection. Drug treatment can fail because of incomplete knowledge regarding innervation, the nature of neurotransmitters, the characteristics of cell receptors and the role of hormonal influences.

Currently, the clinician strives to imitate the action of nerve cells by providing substances which are similar to acetylcholine, norepinephrine or other substances which activate cell receptors. Often, because of ignorance or carelessness, the action of such drugs is negated by the simultaneous use of other medications which are antagonistic (see Chap. XV).

If the detrusor contraction is deficient because of interrupted innervation, bethanacol (Urecholine, Duvoid) is often prescribed to replace the acetylcholine normally released by nerve stimulation. Such replacement can only be effective if there is enough healthy muscle remaining to provide forceful shortening. Furthermore, because of the multiple innervation of the lower tract (see Chap. I), the sphincters may contract, simultaneously opposing the urine outflow. By counteracting sphincter stimulation with the simultaneous administration of the alpha-adrenergic blocker phenoxybenzaline (Dibenzylene), sphincter relaxation is promoted.

Similarly, when sphincter spasticity exists in the presence of normal bladder contraction, phenoxybenzaline can be useful, provided that functional muscle has not been replaced with fibrous connective tissue.

Muscle relaxants such as diazepam (Valium) are often used to relieve spasticity of the external sphincter.

Unfortunately, none of the neuroactive drugs are exclusively selective for the function of the targeted muscles. Consequently, other muscles also innervated by nerves producing cholinergic or adrenergic substances may be affected. In addition, the function of the central nervous system may be adversely influenced, producing undesired side effects.

Surgical intervention is often necessary to prevent the overdistention caused by functional obstruction. Sphincterotomy, the incising of the internal sphincter to enlarge its diameter and prevent its constriction, is a fairly simple procedure. Unfortunately, with existent techniques it results in incontinence and so is not appropriate in females. In some males, scar tissue formation is excessive and repeated sphincterotomies have provided only temporary relief.

In such male patients and in females, the use of an indwelling urethral catheter may prevent inadequate drainage providing that infection can be controlled.

In other cases, none of these therapeutic agents is satisfactory, reflux progresses, kidney tissue is destroyed and renal function declines. In these instances, supravesical diversion is justified. Ileal and colonic diversion have fallen into disrepute because of past misuse or because of the lack of effective instruction of the patient regarding the details of care needed to insure efficient function. When other methods of urinary tract drainage have proven useless, and when instituted before kidney function has declined to levels incompatible with healthful living, diversion can be life saving, permitting the patient to enjoy years of healthful and productive living. In our series of spinal cord injured patients, we have patients with ileal diversion who have been maintained with minimal decline of kidney function for well over fifteen years. However, these patients have been conscientious in self-care and have cooperated with medical supervision so that complications could be corrected if they developed.

AUTONOMIC DYSREFLEXIA

Autonomic dysreflexia is one of the most dangerous syndromes which can affect the quadriplegic or high paraplegic, but it is frequently unrecognized by patients, attendants or health professionals.

The signs and symptoms consist of elevated blood pressure, headache, slow pulse, dilated pupils, and sweating or "goose bumps" above the level of the cord lesion. Not all symptoms are present with every attack, but if the cause is not removed the blood pressure may climb until seizures occur or cerebral hemorrhage results in stroke.

Autonomic dysreflexia is the result of sensory stimulation activating the sympathetic nervous system which has been isolated from the modifying influence of the brain and brain stem by a spinal cord lesion.[8]

In the normal person, sensation is carried to the spinal cord by fibers within a peripheral nerve or accompanying an autonomic nerve. Some of the fibers synapse in the cord with nerve fibers going directly to the sympathetic system, others with fibers going to the brain or brain stem (Fig. XVII-3).

In the intact nervous system, fibers return from the brain or brain stem to the sympathetic system to modify the activity of the stimulated sympathetic nerves. In a spinal cord injured above C6, all the T1 to L2 sympathetic nerve cells receiving sensory stimulation are without any modification from the higher centers and severe reactions may be expected. Injuries between C7 and T6 permit some modulating influences and reactions are generally less intense. Below T6, so much inhibiting effect is received that acute reactions are unlikely.

Although almost any peripheral stimulation may provoke it, the stimuli most likely to initiate autonomic dysreflexia are dilatation of bladder or bowel. It follows that bladder drainage should be checked when autonomic symptoms occur. Has the suprapubic tube slipped out? Has the balloon on the indwelling catheter deflated, permitting the catheter to be extruded? Is the collecting device twisted so that the urinary tract cannot drain? In the appliance-free person, can the bladder be felt above the level of the pubic bone, indicating an outlet obstruction?

If any of these situations exist it must be corrected without delay. Do not "wait until tomorrow" because of the inconvenience of the hour, transportation, or the social calendar. If the bladder cannot be emptied by conventional means, the contents should be removed by suprapubic aspiration.

Autonomic Hyperreflexia

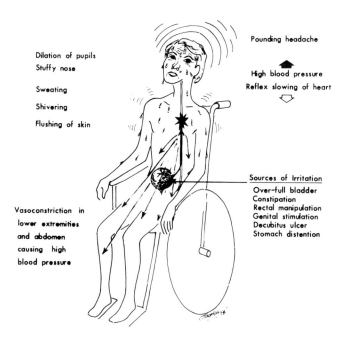

Figure XVII-3. Autonomic dysreflexia.

If the urinary tract is draining, the rectum should be examined and emptied if impacted.

Although the reactions are not usually as severe as those associated with bladder or bowel distention, autonomic symptoms may be the result of burns, frostbite, pressure sores or any other noxious stimulus.

If no cause for the dysreflexia can be found, a sympathetic blocker, such as hydralazine hydrochloride (Apresoline®) or guanethidine (Ismelin®) should be used to decrease the blood pressure. Such measures are seldom necessary, because the cause of hyperreflexia can usually be discovered and removed.

CANCER OF THE BLADDER

Increasing longevity in both able-bodied and disabled people has been accompanied by the problems associated with advancing age. Cancer of the bladder is such an entity. Enumerating the causes of this usually age-related disease is difficult. Contributing factors are not equally prevalent among the population; they tend to appear at different periods of life and they are often synergistic in their actions. Furthermore, setting up analytical studies is hampered by the long-term nature of such investigation. To insure completion of such projects, it is necessary to guarantee continued interest in investigation, procure renewable funding and motivate return to follow-up by patients who find it difficult and expensive.

Since the sixties there has been considerable interest in bladder cancer among the spinal cord injured. However, literature search has not revealed sufficiently long-term studies to provide conclusions, although significant trends have been observed through the data available.

In 1966, Melzak[9] pointed out that in the general population, bladder cancer was twice as prevalent among males as females. Infection was commonly associated as were environmental factors, smoking and bladder stones.

It has been documented that all of these factors are prevelant among the spinal cord injured: males outnumber females, smoking is widespread, urinary tract infection common and bladder stones frequent. Kaufman et al.[10] state that paraplegics have a 16 to 28 times greater than normal risk for squamous cell metaplasia, thought by many to be a precursor to squamous cell cancer. Such metaplasia is often found in patients whose bladders are drained by indwelling catheters.[11] The relative importance of infection, trauma, and foreign body reaction has not been clarified. Cytology and annual cystoscopy have been recommended by many, but Boyarsky[12] advises adding routine, random bladder biopsies because cystoscopic findings may be masked by inflammatory processes. It would be wise to include these procedures in the monitoring of all patients with chronic urinary tract infection.

SUMMARY

The conditions most frequently complicating the long-term care of the disabled bladder are infection, calculi, overdistention, the development of vesicoureteral reflux, episodes of autonomic dysreflexia and cancer of the bladder. In each, prevention is more to be desired than cure. This chapter has endeavored to outline some of the more characteristic signs and symptoms, indicate causes, point out the end results of pathologic progression, and intimate the interrelationship of the various entities. Treatment has been discussed only in general terms because of the rapid obsolescence of specific measures.

M.P.

REFERENCES

1. Scott, R.: Urinary tract stone disease, classic studies. *Urol 6:*667, 1975.
2. Griffith, D., Gibson, J., Clinton, C., and Musher, D.: Acetohydroxamic acid: Clinical studies of a urease inhibitor in patients with staghorn renal calculi. *J Urol 119:*9–15, 1978.
3. Williams, J., Rodman, J., and Peterson, C.: A randomized double-blind study of acetohydroxamic acid in struvite nephrolithiasis. *N Engl J Med 311:*760, 1984.
4. Cox, C., and Hinman, Jr., F.: Experiments with induced bacteriuria, vesical emptying and bacterial growth on the mechanism of bladder defense to infection. *J Urol 86:*739, 1961.
5. Boen, J., and Sylvester, D.: The mathematical relationship among urinary frequency, residual urine, and bacterial growth in bladder infections. *Invest Urol 2:*468, 1964.
6. Boen, J.: A quantitative discussion of the effectiveness of voiding as a defense against bladder infection. *Biometrics 22:*53, 1966.
7. Sperling, K.: unpublished data, Dept. Physical Medicine and Rehabilitation, Univ. of Wisconsin, Madison.
8. Cole, T., Kottke, F., Olson, M., Stradal, L., and Niederloh, J.: Alterations in cardiovascular control in high spinal myelomalacia. *Arch Phys Med Rehabil 48:*359, 1967.
9. Melzak, J.: The incidence of bladder cancer in paraplegia. *Paraplegia 4:*85, 1966.
10. Kaufman, J., Bushra, F., Jacobs, S., Gabilonda, F., Yalla, S., Kane, J., and Rossier, A.: Bladder cancer and squamous metaplasia in spinal cord injury patients. *J Urol 118:*967, 1977.
11. Newman, D., Brown, J., Jay, A., and Pontius, E.: Squamous cell carcinoma of the bladder. *J Urol 100:*470, 1968.
12. Boyarsky, S.: Bladder cancer and spinal cord-injured patients. *Urol 15:*693, 1980.

Chapter XVIII

AGING AND URINARY TRACT DISABILITY

GENERAL EFFECTS OF AGING

Aging affects all parts of the urinary system, the expulsive forces, the uriniferous components, the renal hormones and enzymes affecting hematopoiesis and control of blood pressure, the prostate gland encircling the male urethra and the pelvic sling which holds the bladder in an optimum position, as well as the peripheral and central nervous controls of the urinary tract.

Pathologists and gerontologists are fond of speculating about the relative effects of prolonged age versus the results of the stresses and insults to human physiology occurring in the life of every individual. When we speak of aging, we will refer to the changes, developing over time, which cannot be attributed to trauma or recognized disease entities, bearing in mind that such changes will be superimposed upon the inherent problems of those who also suffer from conditions such as congenital malformations, spinal cord injury, brain damage, diabetes, peripheral neuropathies, demyelinating diseases, stroke, malignancies and a host of other pathologic entities. As skill in dealing with disease increases, the effects of senescence will become increasingly important.

AGING AND THE KIDNEY

Nature has been generous to the developing organism by providing more than twice the amount of kidney tissue necessary to maintain a healthy body. The glomeruli become fully mature between ages four and eight years while the tubules continue maturation until about age eighteen.[1] The development of vascularization probably parallels that of the glomerulus. Although there is great individual variation, degenerative changes in all three components begin to appear near age thirty.

At that time, alterations in thickness and contractility develop in large and middle size arteries, gradually extending to smaller vessels of the kidneys.[2] By age fifty-five, the vascular bed has diminished by about 20 percent. Some of the glomeruli show collapse of the capillaries and later become fibrosed entirely or in part. Some eventually disappear, so that between ages sixty and seventy, many persons have lost one-third to one-half of the original number of glomeruli. Similarly, but to a lesser degree, the tubular component decreases with subsequent polyuria and lowered urinary specific gravity. With the diminution of parenchymal tissue, the fibrillar interstitium compacts and kidney size is reduced.

As a result of these changes, kidney function declines. Shock and his co-workers[3] devised a rule-of-thumb simplification of more complex equations for quick calculation of normal values of kidney function per given age. For glomerular filtration rate (GFR), expected function should equal $130 - (\text{age} - 30)$ ml/min/1.73 M². Tubular function, defined as TmPAH, should equal $100 - (\text{age} - 30)$ mg/min/1.73 M².

In some respects, the aging kidney is less able to compensate for stress than the youthful kidney. Hypertrophy of the parenchymal tissue remaining after loss caused by disease or surgery slows as age advances.[4] On the other hand, anastomotic branching increases within the kidney as atherosclerosis advances.[2] Nevertheless, the net result is decrease in the vascular bed.

The effect of geriatric changes upon renal hormone and enzyme production requires more research. However, it seems probable that aging is responsible for some of the anemias as well as changes in blood pressure control in the elderly.

AGING AND THE BLADDER

Degenerative changes in the bladder occur as smooth muscle and elastic tissue are replaced by fibrous connective tissue. Closure can become inefficient at both ureteral and urethral orifices favoring vesicoureteral reflux and leading to difficulty in closing or opening the bladder outlet. Brocklehorst[5] claims that many instances of slowness in starting the urinary stream are due, in both men and women, to fibrosis of the bladder outlet. In addition, men are subject to obstruction following benign prostatic hypertrophy or prostatic malignancy. Women often become incontinent because of child-birth or surgery which weakens the pelvic musculature and produces a funnel-shaped deformity which prevents the efficient closure of the external sphincter.

An often unrecognized hindrance to normal bladder function in the aged is defective peripheral innervation. Pelvic surgery in women sometimes results in interrupted sensory or motor fibers. In men, prostatic surgery can result in incontinence due to nerve disruption as well as the modification of the sphincter. Functional changes can occur due to alcoholic neuropathy or the neuropathy accompanying late onset diabetes. While such changes are not primarily the result of aging, they become accentuated by passing time.

Development of uninhibited bladder contractions in older people is not well understood but can cause troublesome frequency and precipitancy.

AGING AND THE NERVOUS SYSTEM

As the life span increases, so does the incidence of central nervous system changes. While most elderly people maintain their perceptual abilities, in others sensory awareness diminishes so that increasing urine volume is not recognized until involuntary micturition occurs. Shortened attention span can cause others to forget to complete an effort to get to the toilet facilities. In more extreme cases, there is a lack of concern about the consequences of micturition and defecation. The apparent rise in incidence of Alzheimer's disease, plus our present-day helplessness with regard to its treatment, has accentuated our awareness of these unfortunate conditions.

AGING AND URINARY TRACT INFECTIONS

Even less well understood is the propensity of the aged for urinary tract infections. Perhaps it is due to some breakdown in the always poorly defined defense mechanisms of the bladder. It is very likely that the lessened sensation of thirst after fluid deprivation[6] contributes to the lack of urine dilution and bladder washout. Regardless of etiology, diagnosis of infection is made more difficult by the absence of fever and the reduced recognition of pain which frequently accompanies advancing age.

BEHAVIORAL APPROACH TO INCONTINENCE

How can problems of urinary tract changes in the elderly be approached so that renal deterioration does not occur? High quality medical and surgical management is important when indicated, but it can often be obviated if behavioral changes are instituted. Intake of fluids even in the absence of thirst can be bolstered by increasing the fluid content of foods served at meals and at snack times. Soups, stews, gelatins, custards, ice cream and sherbets at meal time, decaffeinated drinks, bouillons, iced tea, fruit juices, milk shakes and frozen deserts at snack times can augment the water intake which is so often resisted.

Incontinence can often be avoided by establishing and enforcing a time schedule for voiding using shorter time intervals to accommodate the smaller bladder capacities often found in the aged. In those with lessened mentation, it may be necessary to determine individual behavior patterns which provide cues to the full bladder: discomfort may be evinced by nervousness, apprehension, manual pressure of the meatus or "wandering" behavior.

Infection must be suspected if incontinence increases, the skin of perineum or upper thighs becomes red and irritated, or if the urine has a foul odor. Recording the individual's normal temperature so that a temperature deviation can be reported in degrees may aid in convincing reluctant physicians or health care supervisors that urine cultures are necessary.

THE EFFECT OF AGING ON OTHER DISABILITIES

The viscissitudes of aging add to the problems in caring for other disabling conditions and will become increasingly important as improving care of the disabled results in greater longevity. In stroke patients, there is often increasing forgetfulness and poor judgement. With brain damage, spinal cord lesions and multiple sclerosis, there are added sensory and motor deficits resulting in over- or under-activity of the bladder. In the neuropathies and other systemic or neurologic disorders, there may be increased involvement of renal or bladder function due directly to changes in innervation, or indirectly to changes in hormonal or catecholamine production.

The province of this book is not to deal with the specifics of care for every pathological entity. However, it is the hope of the authors that the principles here presented will aid in the development of care plans through the recognition of the signs and symptoms of urinary tract dysfunction and careful monitoring of treatment while remaining aware of the dangers in all kinds of urinary tract drainage.

M.P.

REFERENCES

1. Darmady, E., Offer, J., and Woodhouse, M.: The parameters of the aging kidney. *J Pathol 109:*195, 1972.
2. Dock, W.: The decrease in vascularity of human hearts and kidneys between the third and sixth decades. *Science 93:*349, 1941.
3. Watkin, J., and Schock, N.: Agewise standard value for CIn, CPAH and TmPAH. *Am Soc Clin Invest 341:*969, 1970.
4. Oliver, J.: Problems of aging. In *Urinary System.* Baltimore, Williams and Wilkins, 1952.
5. Brockelhorst, J.: Aging of the human bladder. *Geriatrics 21:*154, 1972.
6. Phillips, P., Rolls, B., Ledingham, J., Forsling, M., Morton, J., Crowe, M., and Wollner, L.: Reduced thirst after water deprivation in healthy elderly men. *N Eng J Med 311:*753, 1984.

Chapter XIX

THE ROLE OF ALLIED HEALTH CARE PROFESSIONALS IN URINARY TRACT CARE

The role of physicians and nurses in long-term urinary care is well established. It is hoped that the information included in this book will be of value to them in their care of patients. Perhaps less well known is the role of other health care professionals. Many often become involved in the care of patients with long-term disabilities who also have long-term urinary problems. It is the responsibility of each health care professional to be aware of the different methods of urinary drainage, to help prevent urinary tract trauma and infection and to minimize patient embarrassment, making use of every opportunity to monitor conditions and to help motivate the patients to assume responsibility for their own care.

The roles played and the opportunities for intervention will vary with disciplines, but some general recommendations apply to all.

1. Know the method of urinary drainage used by the patient. Care procedures will differ with each method of drainage. Be aware of these differences so information given to the patient will be accurately reinforced and patient motivation encouraged.

2. If urinary appliances are used, know where they are positioned. Care must be taken when transferring or transporting patients to ensure that the catheter or tubing is not caught on the arm of the wheelchair or other objects and that the patient is not positioned on top of the appliance or tubing. Seat belts and clothing should not be put on in a manner that will obstruct urine flow (see Chap. XI, "Positioning of Urinary Drainage Equipment").

3. Know the patient's fluid intake requirements. Patients who are on an intermittent catheterization program usually are on a more rigidly controlled fluid intake program in order to regulate their catheterization schedules. Patients who use an indwelling urethral or suprapubic catheter should be consistently drinking more fluids to help keep bacteria washed out of their bladder. Offering these patients a glass of water at appropriate times will help to emphasize the need for good fluid intake as well as provide the opportunity for it. Water and cranberry juice are the best fluids

to offer patients, as citrus fruit juices, soda pops and fruit-ades tend to alkalinize the urine (see Chap. V, "Effect of Diet and Fluid Intake").

4. Be aware of the patient's daily urinary tract care schedule. If the patient is on an intermittent catheterization program and it is time to be catheterized, this should take precedence over other appointments. By encouraging conformance to schedules, you are reinforcing the importance of proper timing to avoid bladder overdistention.

5. Be aware of the patient's medication schedule. Many medications are most effective when given on a regular schedule. Adjust your appointments to accommodate this schedule. If a patient is on a self-medication program and wishes to take medications in your presence, know what is being taken and be sure it is taken in the prescribed manner. Some medication should be taken with milk or food, while others should be taken when the stomach is empty. Some medications should not be taken with other drugs. The health care professional's concern will help to reinforce the need to follow instructions closely.

6. Be prepared to deal with problems that may develop while the patient is in your care. What should be done if the patient has a full leg bag? How and where can it be emptied? A clean receptacle, non-sterile gloves and alcohol wipes should be available for your own protection as well as the patient's. Put on gloves. Wipe emptying spout with alcohol wipes and empty the urine into receptacle. Wipe the spout with alcohol. Wipe to remove any remaining drops of urine and reclamp or cap the spout. Empty and rinse the receptacle in the proper place. This receptacle is now contaminated; dispose of it properly. Remove gloves and wash hands. Again, remember you are setting an example for the patient. Teach the proper procedure.

What should be done if the catheter and tubing become separated and urine spills? If a clamp or forcep is available, clamp off the catheter to prevent further leakage. Put on non-sterile gloves. Vigorously wipe the end of the catheter and the end of the tubing with alcohol, reconnect the tubing and catheter and unclamp. Clean up all the spilled urine with a suitable disinfectant or alcohol. Sponge clothing, if wet, with alcohol. Clean up any urine spilled on furniture or floor.

What should be done if the patient develops autonomic hyperreflexia? Be aware of the symptoms which may include a severe headache of rapid onset, sweating, dilated pupils, shivering, goose bumps, and flushing of the skin. Many of these symptoms are produced by an increase in blood pressure and the condition can be life threatening. See Chapter XVII for a more complete discussion of autonomic hyperreflexia. If the condition is suspected, look for the cause and eliminate it, if possible. Autonomic hyperreflexia is frequently brought on by a full bladder which may have resulted from a full leg bag, the need for catheterization, or kinked or plugged catheter or tubing. Other things that may lead to the condition are: a full rectum, pressure areas, or any condition which would be felt as pain by a person with normal sensation. If the cause cannot be found and eliminated, the patient should be placed in an upright sitting position, which should reduce the headache somewhat, and a physician notified.

It is extremely important to be aware of the function of the different types of urinary drainage appliances and the dangers associated with each method. A review of the material presented in Chapters V through XI will provide information about each method of drainage and care procedures. How well the health care professional is informed and handles emergencies will have an impact on the patients.

7. Be aware that the patients may be struggling with adjustment to changes in body image. Be sensitive to their feelings. Provide privacy when emptying leg bags, working with their urinary drainage equipment or discussing urinary problems.

8. If you are called upon to assist in teaching urinary tract care procedures to family members, friends or attendants, it is important that you know the details of correct procedures. Don't give out misinformation.

NURSES

The role of nurses in urinary tract care has been addressed throughout this book. It is perhaps good to re-emphasize the importance of consistency in care and teaching. Remember, the patients will learn by what they see as well as by what they hear or read. Good teaching and training is ineffective if health care professionals do not follow the advocated procedure.

Develop good urinary tract care procedures and protocols for your facility and then be sure they are followed. Develop patient and family education training programs consistent with the procedures used in your facility.

Continuity of care after discharge is important. If the patient is to be followed by a public health or home nursing care service, that agency should be informed of the procedures and protocols in use with the patient. Equally as important as establishing a good teaching relationship with nursing care professionals is the establishment of a working relationship with out-of-hospital physicians involved in the care of the patient. This contact is valued by most physicians, especially if it is done in a tactful manner.

School nurses have in the past occasionally been called upon to help a student with urinary problems. The current trend of including children with disabilities in the regular school system is increasing the number of students with long-term urinary problems and presenting a challenge to the health care professionals. It is sometimes difficult for these students to adjust to the school environment. A means of tending to urinary cares with privacy will have to be provided.

Children on intermittent catheterization programs will probably need to be catheterized at some time during the school day. Appropriate facilities should be furnished. The catheterization procedures used by children may vary considerably and may be in conflict with the procedures considered by the nurse to be most appropriate. It is recommended that a procedure for a student's urinary tract care be discussed with the student, the parents and their physicians. It is sometimes advisable (to avoid future legal problems) to also include the school attorney.

OCCUPATIONAL AND PHYSICAL THERAPISTS

The disciplines of physical and occupational therapy have been combined for discussion here because their roles may vary considerably in different settings, with duties frequently overlapping. The therapists have an exceptional opportunity to work with a patient on a one-to-one basis for long periods of time. Consequently, a knowledgeable therapist can *monitor* and help *motivate* patients to *maintain* good urinary tract care. In addition to the previously listed concerns, the therapist may find all or some of the following apply.

Range of Motion, Exercise and Other Activities

The urine collecting appliance (leg bag, night bag, jug) should always be kept below the level of the bladder, even during dressing exercises and other activities. If the patient is wearing a leg bag during lower extremity activities, the tubing should be clamped close to the catheter, external catheter or ostomy pouch, or the leg bag removed from the leg and placed on the bed or mat. This will prevent urine in the leg bag or tubing from running back towards the bladder (see Chap. XI, "Positioning Urinary Drainage Equipment"). Generally, the tubing can be clamped for periods of twenty to thirty minutes without resulting in bladder overdistention. If the patient has a high urine output and small capacity bladder, it may be necessary to position the collecting appliance below the level of the bladder and unclamp at periodic intervals so that the bladder may empty. BE SURE TO UNCLAMP THE TUBING WHEN ACTIVITY IS COMPLETED.

Whirlpools, Tanks, and Tubs

When placing a patient with a urinary appliance into a whirlpool, tank or tub, clamp the tubing close to the catheter, external catheter or ostomy pouch and place the leg bag or night bag over the edge of the tank or tub (see Chap. XI, "Positioning of Urinary Drainage Equipment"). This will prevent urine from flowing back towards the bladder. BE SURE TO UNCLAMP THE TUBING WHEN THE ACTIVITY IS COMPLETED. Again, if the patients are to be in the water for long periods of time, it may be necessary at periodic intervals to raise them up so the collecting appliance is below the level of the bladder, unclamp the tubing and allow the bladder to empty.

Discuss urinary tract management with the patient. Be aware of their urinary tract care needs, offer fluids when appropriate, and provide an opportunity to empty urine collecting appliances if necessary. Remember, you are setting an example for the patient by your interest and concern, and by the way you handle their appliances.

Supplies and Literature

In many health care facilities it is the occupational or physical therapist who provides the patients with the necessary urinary drainage supplies and/or information regarding sources of these supplies, so it is important to keep up to date on the latest equipment and current sources.

Adaptive Equipment

Adaptive equipment is often necessary to help patients attain the maximum degree of independence. Therapists should be aware of the dangers associated with each method of urinary drainage so equipment is designed that will not compromise the integrity of the drainage system (see Chapters V–XI).

Proper placement of the leg bag is essential to good urinary drainage. The leg bag should be placed below the knee so that it is below the level of the bladder when the patient is in a seated position. Frequently, it is difficult to maintain the leg bag in this position without fastening the straps so tight that there is danger of impaired circulation. The therapist should be able to develop a strap mechanism that will be suitable for each individual patient; one example is shown in Figure XIX-1. Double straps with Velcro are used, with one placed above the knee and one below the knee. The two straps are joined at the side by a short strap. Buttons on the lower strap permit easy attachment of the leg bag. The strap above the knee will prevent the bag from sliding down the leg.

Velcro straps with appropriate loops are usually easier to use for patients with decreased finger dexterity than the rubber straps provided with most leg bags.

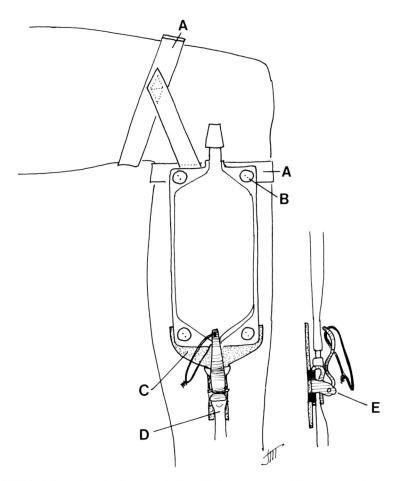

Figure XIX-1. Adaptations for leg bag. A. Double leg bag strap with one strap above the knee and one strap below the knee. B. Buttons on strap for attaching leg bag. C. Backboard to help stabilize tubing. D. Drainage tubing with clamp attached. E. Side view of clamp showing a cord loop to assist in opening clamp.

Also of importance is a safe convenient emptying spout. A short piece of tubing attached to the bottom of the bag, closed with a clamp, is often easier for a patient to manage than the cap provided with many leg bags. The clamp may have a loop attached to it for easier grasping. A small backboard of plastic or fiberboard will help stabilize the tubing (Fig. XIX-1).

These and other adaptations may help the patient develop a greater degree of independence. Be sure the system you develop will not lead to urinary problems for the patient (e.g. increased urinary tract infections).

A therapist may also be called upon to develop methods for attaching urine collecting bags or jugs to wheelchairs or beds. Hooks, pouches and tapes attached to the wheelchair or bed are often used. Adhesive-backed Velcro strips can be attached under the wheelchair and used to help suspend the tubing (Fig. XIX-2). Keep in mind when developing these assistive devices that the jug or bag should always be kept below the level of the bladder with the tubing in as straight a descending line as possible.

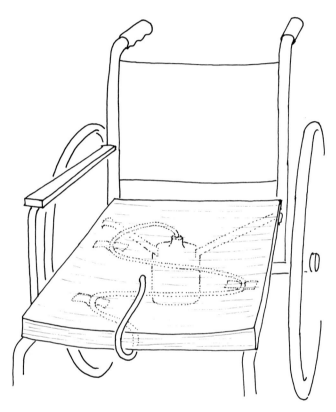

Figure XIX-2. Attachment of urine collecting appliance with long tubing (e.g. night bag) under a wheelchair. Adhesive backed Velcro (hook) strips are placed on underside of chair seat. The tubing is anchored to these strips with pieces of Velcro (loop) tape.

Seat Belts and Clothing

Obstruction of urine flow by clothing or seat belts that are too tight must be avoided. It is sometimes necessary to cut a hole in a corset or abdominal binder to accommodate an ostomy bag. Occasionally, padding with foam strips will eliminate pressure on an ostomy appliance or catheter (see Chap. X, "Body Support Garments"). Zippers or Velcro strips placed in clothing in appropriate places will often be an aid in urinary care procedures by providing easier access.

Knowing the dangers will help guide the therapist when making adaptations. Knowing the patient's fluid intake schedule will enable the therapist to provide water at appropriate times. When working with patients, the therapist should check the patient's urine collecting devices and provide an opportunity to empty them if necessary. Setting a good example by interest and concern for correct procedures will help to motivate the patient to do likewise.

PSYCHOLOGISTS AND SOCIAL WORKERS

Although psychologists and social workers do not treat the physical aspects of disability directly, it is important that they be aware of the patient's urinary status, including the method of urinary drainage in use.

As with other disciplines, ask your patient about fluid intake, catheterization and urinary care schedules. Provide opportunities to empty appliances and obtain fluids to drink. A direct approach will help establish the importance of schedules. Psychologists and social workers can play an active role in helping patients adjust to changes in body image resulting from the use of urinary drainage appliances. They need someone with whom to discuss their feelings in their effort to re-establish their self-esteem. It is important then to be aware of the method of drainage in use, the dangers, and basic care procedures to better understand the concerns of the patient. Asking the patient questions about catheterization and medication schedules and providing opportunities to empty leg bags and obtain fluids at the proper time will not only help establish the importance of these schedules and procedures but also provide an opportunity for the patient to discuss some of their feelings related to their changed urinary status.

Some patients, because of their physical or psychosocial problems, are not motivated to learn about or participate in their care procedures. The psychologist or social worker can help the other health professionals develop more effective methods of working with these patients. This type of information is often transmitted through regular team meetings if the team approach to care is being used in the facility. If this method is not formally utilized, direct contact with each health care professional involved in the patient's care should be made to discuss the best methods to help the patient attain goals and maintain maximal health.

OTHERS

All persons involved with the care of patients having long-term urinary drainage problems should have a basic understanding of the methods of urinary drainage and know what to do if problems arise. This includes x-ray technicians, transport carriers, orderlies, nursing aides, personal attendants, and family members.

Improper placement of urinary drainage appliances during transport, transfers, x-rays and other activities may allow backflow of urine, cause an appliance to be pulled or other dangerous conditions to occur.

Nursing aids, attendants and family members who are actively involved in patient care can have a great influence on the patient by using proper procedures and encouraging compliance to schedules and procedures. Assertiveness on the part of the attendant or family member and open communication with the patient will often identify problems. A clearly stated problem can more rationally be treated than a vague expression and may prevent serious problems from developing.

APPENDICES

Appendix I

ACID–ALKALINE ASH DIET

ACID ASH DIET

Suggested Foods You Should Eat to Keep Your Urine Acid:

A. Soups and Juices
> Bouillon
> Meat broths
> Soups made with foods allowed
> Prune juice
> Plum juice
> Cranberry juice

B. Meat, Fish, and Poultry
> At least two large servings of any kind, especially chicken, duck, and lean beef.

C. Eggs
> One or more in any form.

D. Dairy Products
> Not more than 1 pint of milk and 3 ounces of soft cheese, especially cottage cheese, cream cheese, Gruyere, Gorgonzola, Cheddar, and Swiss.

E. Vegetables
> Three small servings of any vegetable except those not allowed. Corn, white beans, and lentils may be used freely.

F. Potato Substitutes
> Two or more servings of white or brown rice, noodles, macaroni, spaghetti, or barley.

G. Fruits
> Two small servings of any fruit except those not allowed. Prunes, plums, and cranberries may be used freely.

H. Salads
> Any fruit or vegetable salad made with the food allowed, served with oil and vinegar dressing.

I. Cereals

One or more servings, dry or cooked, preferably whole grain or enriched.

J. Breads

Four or more slices, preferably whole grain or enriched. Crackers, if salt is not restricted.

K. Desserts

Cake (without fruit)   Plum tarts
Prune whip   Jello®
Rice custard   Bread pudding
Cookies   Cornstarch pudding
Tapioca pudding   Custard pie

L. Beverages

Coffee (decaffeinated)
Tea (herbal)

M. Concentrated Sweets

White sugar
Corn syrup
Cranberry sauce
Plum jelly
Candy other than chocolate with almonds

N. Concentrated Fats

Butter   Oil
Nut butter   Olive oil
Cooking fats   Mayonnaise made with
                                vinegar

O. Miscellaneous

Peanuts   Walnuts
Filberts   Brazil nuts

ALKALINE ASH DIET

Foods You Should Avoid in Excess Amounts to Keep Your Urine Acid

A. Juices

Citrus fruit juices such as orange, lemon, lime, and tomato.

B. Dairy Products

   Avoid excessive amounts of milk products including malts and milk shakes.

C. Vegetables

Potatos	Lima beans
Soy beans	Beet greens
Parsnips	Spinach
Dried vegetables	Tomatoes

D. Fruits

Cantaloupe	Raisins
Dates	Figs
Citrus fruits	Dried fruits (except prunes)

E. Beverages

   Flavored sodas
   Fruit-ades

F. Miscellaneous

Olives	Molasses
Almonds	Chestnuts
Coconut	

Appendix II

MODERATE LOW SODIUM DIET

NO ADDED SALT AND NO SALTY FOODS DIET

This diet allows a minimal amount of salt in cooking, avoiding all highly salted foods and eliminating all use of salt at the table. No special foods are needed for this diet. Foods may be prepared the same as usual, however, do not add salt at the table. Garlic powder and onion powder may be used but not garlic salt or onion salt. Commercial salad dressings should be used in moderation.

Foods and Condiments to Avoid:

A. Seasonings

Salt	Steak sauces
Celery salt	Worcestershire sauce
Popcorn salt	Kitchen Bouquet®
Garlic salt	Chili sauce
Onion salt	Catsup*
Meat tenderizers	Mustard
Monosodium glutamate	Soy sauce

B. Snacks

Pretzels	Corn curls	Pickles
Potato chips	Cheese curls	Olives
Salted crackers	Salted popcorn	Salted snack foods
Salted nuts		

C. Smoked, Cured or Fried Meats, Fish, and Cheese

Ham	Sausage	Frankfurters
Luncheon meat	Pastrami	Canned meat and fish
Bacon	Cheese spreads	Smoked meat, fish,
Corned beef	Sardines	and fowl
Dried beef	Kosher meats	Processed cheese
Anchovies	Caviar	Salt pork
Pickled herring		

---

*Salt-free catsup is available.

D. Miscellaneous

Canned soups   Foods in a brine
Broth or bouillon cubes   Sauerkraut
Packaged and frozen main dishes   Pizza
Buttermilk

TRIAL OF VOIDING

Pre-admission

1. Laboratory work
   a. Urine culture
   b. Antibiotic sensitivities
   c. Antibody coated bacteria determination
   d. Cystogram for reflux
   e. Intravenous pyelogram
2. Give appropriate antibiotics
   a. 2 days before trial.
   b. Plan to continue during and at least 3 days after trial.
3. Have PATIENT keep accurate records of fluid intake and output before trial.
4. Explain entire procedure to patient.
   a. Records he/she must keep
      1. Intake
      2. Spontaneous output
      3. Triggered output
      4. Residual urine.
   b. Protocol
5. Prepare patient psychologically.
   a. Probable initial failure.
   b. If there is no success in reasonable period of time, will have another chance later.
6. Do not schedule therapy during trial.
7. Supervising physician must be available during trial.

PROTOCOL FOR TRIAL OF VOIDING

A. *First Day*
   1. Physician(s), accompanied by involved nursing staff
      a. Review
         1. Records to be kept
         2. Protocol

  b. Show patient
    1. Conventional gas cystometer tracing
    2. Educational gas cystometrogram
        a. Introduce 200 ml gas in bladder
        b. Shut off gas inflow
        c. Leave chart moving
        d. Physician to go through all methods of bladder stimulation, letting patient see relative efficiency by watching the chart:
            1. Tapping
            2. Crede
            3. Crede with bending
            4. Straining
            5. Digital anal stimulation
            6. Hair pulling
            7. Thigh stroking
            8. Other.
        e. Patient repeats all maneuvers, watching tracing
B. Physician—remove catheter.
C. Patient records time.
D. Physician arranges that patient drinks 200 ml every 60 minutes and records time and amount of intake.
E. Patient records time and amount of spontaneous voiding. (He/she may need help in estimating amount.)
F. In two hours doctor supervises stimulating for voiding. If possible, patient does the stimulating.
G. Amount of triggered voiding is measured; patient records.
H. Physician measures residual; patient records.
I. *Subsequent efforts (first day)*
    1. If patient is tired or staff cannot be present, leave catheter in place and set time for next effort.
    2. Otherwise, remove catheter, record time and repeat effort.
    3. Try to have at least three trials the first day.
    4. If residual after last trial is *greater than 50 ml*, leave catheter in place until following morning, having patient record intake and output.
    5. If residual is less than 50 ml, leave catheter out until bedtime, stimulating bladder every two hours and recording output.
    6. At bedtime stimulate bladder, replace catheter, measure residual and leave catheter in all night.
J. *Second Day*
    1. Physician reviews records and determines amount of fluid intake and intervals between drinking.

2. Reinforce patient psychologically.
3. Follow previous day's protocol.
4. If last residual small and patient is not a night voider, leave catheter out, limit fluids, and leave written orders for times of stimulation during night.

K. *Successive Days*

1. Physician reviews previous records and leaves written orders for day's protocol.

L. If trial is successful (residual consistently near 50 ml or less)

1. Arrange for additional antibiotics.
2. Arrange for residual measurement with cultures:
   a. twice weekly for one week.
   b. once a week for two weeks.
   c. every two weeks for one month.
   d. once a month for three months
   e. every three months for six months
   f. every six months indefinitely.

TECHNIQUES USED IN MULTIPLE EFFORT TRIAL OF VOIDING

Credé

1. With the hand flat and held parallel to a line connecting the two anterior superior iliac spines, sweep down from above the umbilicus toward the symphysis pubis, increasing pressure as you approach the symphysis and exerting as much pressure as possible just above this bone.
2. Draw your fist from above the umbilicus toward the symphysis, increasing pressure until you are pressing very hard against the bladder.

Credé with Bending

Credé with fist. Push hard against the bladder and have the patient bend forward as hard as possible over fist.

Tapping

Use dominant hand to provide both strength and endurance. Results will depend upon sensitivity of bladder to mechanical stimulation (jarring). Strike the area over the bladder with the ulnar edge of the hand (anatomical medial—i.e. the side with the fifth finger). First, use gentle tapping for at least 30 seconds. If still no results, tap with all your strength for at least 60 seconds. (This is very tiring. Practice to build up your endurance.)

Digital Stimulation

With gloved, lubricated finger in the anus, press first with a circular motion. If there is no bladder contraction, move finger from side to side. If still no contraction, slowly, but firmly move "around the clock," exerting pressure at each "numeral." If any of these maneuvers produce bladder contraction, record successful area(s), e.g. 2 o'clock or 3 and 9 o'clock.

Thigh Stroking

Stroke medial aspect of thigh, starting close to the genitalia. Usually, a light stroking is more effective than a heavy one.

Hair Pulling

Pulling the pubic hair. Practice on yourself to see how hard hair must be pulled to cause mild pain. With the patient, continue this at least 30 seconds before giving up.

GLOSSARY

ABDOMINAL PADS: absorbent pads designed for abdominal surgery but used for many purposes.

ACID ASH: food or drink which acidifies the urine.

ACIDOSIS: lowered blood bicarbonate.

ACUTE: describing a disease or symptoms of abrupt onset, or lasting a short period of time.

ADENOCARCINOMA: a malignant tumor of gland cells.

ADHESION: the attraction existing between surfaces.

ADVENTITIA: connective tissue layer surrounding organs and connecting them to adjacent organs.

AEROBE: a microorganism which can live and grow in the presence of free oxygen.

AFFERENT: leading toward a structure, often the spinal cord.

AFFERENT ARTERIOLE: small arterial vessel which supplies blood to the kidney glomerulus.

AGAR: a substance upon which bacteria may grow.

ALDOSTERONE: a hormone of the adrenal cortex which causes reabsorption of salt by the kidney distal tubule.

ALPHA ADRENERGIC: receptors on smooth muscle which respond to neuro-transmitters and cause contraction.

ALKALINE ASH: food or drink which alkalinizes the urine.

AMBULATORY: walking.

AMELIORATION: lessening, or making more nearly optimal.

AMINOGLYCOSIDES: a class of antibiotic.

AMYLOID: an abnormal protein deposit in various organs or tissues.

ANAEROBE: a microorganism able to live without air or free oxygen.

ANASTOMOSIS: a connection between tubular structures (as between blood vessels).

ANEURISM: a sac-like bulging of a blood vessel (usually an artery).

ANTIBODIES: proteins synthesized by the body (lymphocytes) to combat foreign substances.

ANTIDIURETIC: suppressing the secretion of urine.

ANTIDIURETIC HORMONE: a hormone released by the posterior pituitary gland which causes the renal medulla to concentrate urine by reabsorbing water from the urine.

AORTA: principle arterial vessel of the body. It receives blood from the heart for distribution to the rest of the body.

APEX/APICES: tip, or pointed end of a conical structure.

293

ARCUATE: arch shaped.

ARTERY: muscular tubes (vessels) that carry oxygenated blood away from the heart and to the tissues of the body.

ASEPTO SYRINGE: large glass or plastic syringe powered by a squeezable rubber bulb.

ASYMMETRIC: disproportion between two or more like parts.

ATONY: lack of muscle tone or strength.

ATROPHY: wasting; progressive degeneration and loss of function.

ATYPICAL: differing from normal.

AUTOPHAGIA: the breakdown (digestion) by a cell of its own aged organelles.

AUTONOMIC DYSREFLEXIA: inappropriate response of the autonomic nervous system characterized by an excessive rise in blood pressure and other symptoms.

AUTONOMIC NERVOUS SYSTEM: adjusts and coordinates vital visceral activities such as digestion, body temperature and blood pressure. Consists of two main divisions, sympathetic and parasympathetic.

AUTONOMIC NEUROGENIC BLADDER: the result of nerve lesion above spinal cord segments S2, 3 and 4. The bladder empties reflexly and often incompletely.

AUTONOMOUS NEUROGENIC BLADDER: the result of nerve lesion at spinal cord segments S2, 3 and 4, or of the peripheral nerves arising from those segments. The bladder does not contract and becomes distended. Urine is released only by overflow.

BACTERICIDAL: causing death of bacteria.

BACTERIOPHAGE: viruses that parasitize bacteria.

BACTERIOSTATIC: inhibiting growth or reproduction of bacteria.

BACTERURIA: bacteria present in the urine.

BARORECEPTOR: sensory nerve endings which respond to pressure.

BENIGN: mild; non-malignant.

BETA ADRENERGIC: receptors on smooth muscle which respond to neurotransmitters to cause relaxation.

BIOPSY: examination of living tissue removed from the body.

BLADDER (vesicle): hollow muscular organ which serves as a reservoir for urine.

BLADDER OUTLET: aperture in the base of the bladder where it opens into the urethra.

BLOCKAGE: use of a chemical to fill receptor sites so that a neurotransmitter is blocked from having an effect on the cell.

BLOOD PLASMA: the fluid part of blood minus the blood cells.

BOLUS: a volume of material forming a single unit in a fluid channel.

BROWNIAN MOVEMENT: motion of minute particles suspended in a liquid.

CALCULUS: "stone"; an abnormal stony concretion formed of mineral salts.

CALYCEAL BLUNTING: rounding of the profile of the fornix due to increased back pressure on the papilla.

CALYX/CALYCES: cup-shaped subdivision of renal pelvis enclosing the apex of the medullary pyramid. Urine drips from the collecting ducts into the calyx.

CAPILLARY: smallest blood vessel whose walls are only one cell thick.

CAPSULE: connective tissue covering an organ.

CASTS: red or white cells, epithelial or fat cells, or cellular debris, which has been extruded from the renal tubules, maintaining the general shape of the tubules.

CATECHOLAMINES: compounds which have sympathomimetic activity; neuro-transmitters and hormones of the adrenal gland.

CAUDAD: toward the "tail"; away from the head.

CELLULE: a small compartment; an evagination of bladder wall due to increased intravesical pressure.

CEPHALAD: toward the head.

CHROMOSOME: a unit within a cell nucleus composed of genetic material (genes).

CHRONIC: denoting a long-lasting disease of slow progression.

CHUX®: brand name of large thin pad that is absorbent on one side and waterproofed on the other.

CILIA: minute hair-like protrusions of cell surfaces which are capable of movement.

CLEARANCE: the removal from the blood of a specific substance by the kidney.

CLITORIS: small cylindical erectile body situated at the anterior part of the vulva; the female homologue of the penis.

COAGULATION: the process of blood clot formation.

COCCUS: a berry-shaped microorganism.

COHESION: a force which causes various particles to unite.

CONCAVE: a hollowed surface.

CONDOM: a sheath or cover for the penis.

CONDUIT: artificially formed tube-like structure carrying urine from ureters to outside, e.g. ileal conduit.

CONTINENCE: voluntary control (inhibition) of urination.

CONTRAINDICATION: any condition which renders some particular line of treatment undesirable or improper.

CORTEX: peripheral portion of an organ; outer layer.

CREDÉ: originally an obstetrical technique, this maneuver is used to empty the bladder by applying pressure below the umbilicus and sweeping the hand or fist toward the pubic symphysis.

CYST: an abnormal sac (within the body) containing air or fluid.

CYSTITIS: inflammation of the bladder.

CYSTOGRAPHY: X-raying bladder after injecting radiopaque dye.

CYSTOMETRY: measuring pressures within the bladder.

CYSTOPLASTY: reconstructive surgery on the bladder.

CYSTOSCOPY: examination of the inside of the bladder with a cystoscope.

CYTOPLASM: the substance (protoplasm) of a cell.

DEHISCENSE: act or process of splitting.

DEHYDRATION: removal of water from the body or tissues.

DENERVATION: loss of nerve supply

DENUDEMENT: removal of epithelial covering.

DESQUAMATION: shedding of epithelial cells.

DETRITUS: debris.

DETRUSOR: smooth muscle of the urinary bladder, which, when it contracts, expels the urine.

DIABETES INSIPIDUS: disorder characterized by production of large amounts of dilute urine but no loss of sugar. It is due to lack of normal amounts of antidiuretic hormone.

DIFFERENTIATED: developed into specialized tissue or organ (from an early form).

DISCOID: disk-shaped.

DISTAL: farthest from the point of reference, e.g. the hand is distal to the shoulder; the tip of the catheter is distal to the inserting hand.

DIURESIS: excretion of increased amounts of urine.

DIVERTICULUM: a pouch or sac opening from a tubular or sacular organ.

DUCTUS DEFERENS: male duct from testis and epididymus to the urethra through which sperm travel to reach the outside.

DYSCRASIA, BLOOD: an abnormal state of the blood or its constituents.

DYSSYNERGIA: failure of bladder-emptying contractions to coordinate with inhibition of the external sphincter contractions. This results in the inability to pass urine.

EDEMA: collection of excessive fluid in extracellular (interstitial) spaces, usually causing swelling.

EFFERENT: traveling away from; the motor nerves which leave the spinal cord are called efferent nerves.

EFFERENT ARTERIOLE: small arterial vessel which drains the glomerulus.

ENDOSCOPE: an instrument used to examine the interior of hollow organs or the abdominal cavity.

ENDOTHELIAL CELLS: cells which form the lining of the blood and lymphatic vessels.

ENUCLEATE: to remove whole and clean; to "shell out."

ENZYME: a protein secreted by the body which promotes or accelerates chemical change in other substances.

EPIDEMIOLOGY: science dealing with the relationships of various factors which determine the frequency and distribution of an infectious process (disease).

EPIDIDYMITIS: inflammation of the epididymis.

EPIDIDYMIS: coiled tubule leading from the testis.

EPITHELIUM: a non-vascular layer of cells covering the external or internal surfaces of the body and including the glands derived from these cells.

ERYTHEMA: a morbid redness of the skin.

ETIOLOGY: cause of disease or abnormal condition.

EXCORIATE: to wear off the skin, often by friction or scratching.

EXOGENOUS: growing or originating outside an organism.

EXTRACELLULAR: outside of the cell.

EXTRANEOUS: existing or belonging outside an organism.

EXTRAPERITONEAL: outside the peritoneum (lining of the abdominal cavity).

EXTRAVASATE: blood or other substances released.

EXTROPHY: congenital malformation and turning out of an organ as the bladder.

EXUDATE: a substance deposited in or on a tissue by a vital process or disease.

FACULTATIVE: a microorganism which usually lives in oxygen but can live without free oxygen.

FALSE PASSAGE: unnatural tunnel created by faulty insertion of catheter.

FASCIA: sheet of connective tissue enveloping muscles or organs and underlying skin.

FASTIDIOUS: having complex nutritional requirements.

FENESTRAE: small openings in endothelial cells which permit easy passage of fluid and ions.

FENESTRATED: pierced with one or more openings.

FENESTRATED DRAPE: a piece of fabric or paper with an opening cut in it.

FIBROSIS: the formation of excess fibrous tissue, denoting a degenerative process.

FILAMENT: thread-like structure.

FILTRATION: passing a liquid through a porous mass which prevents substances above a given size from passing.

FISSURE: cleft; groove; slit.

FISTULA: a deep sinous ulcer often leading to an internal organ.

FLAGELLA: elongated thread-like, motile appendages.

FLANK PAIN: pain over side of body between ribs and pelvis.

FLORA: plant, or bacterial growth present in or characteristic of a special location.

FORNIX/FORNICES: the space created by the arching structure of the calyx surrounding the papilla.

FREQUENCY: sensation of the need to urinate at abnormally close intervals.

GANGLION: a collection of nerve cell bodies outside the central nervous system.

GENITALIA (external): reproductive organs lying outside the body.

GLANS: bulbous, distal end of penis.

GLAUCOMA: disease of the eye marked by increased internal pressure.

GLOMERULAR FILTRATION RATE: the amount of fluid that is filtered by the kidney glomeruli per minute.

GLOMERULUS: a small tuft of capillaries in the kidney.

HEMATURIA: blood in the urine.

HELIX: coil.

HEMATOPOESIS: formation of the elements of blood.

HEMOLYTIC: able to destroy (lyse) red blood cells.

HERNIATE: forceful protrusion through a wall or membrane.

HIATUS: an opening, aperture, or fissure.

HOMOLOGUE: an organ similar in structure, position, and origin to another organ.

HORMONE: a chemical messenger formed by a gland and carried by the blood to act on another "target" organ.

HYDRODYNAMICALLY: relating to the force of fluids acting on solid bodies immersed in fluid.

HYDRONEPHROSIS: dilatation of pelvis and calyces resulting from obstruction to the flow of urine.

HYDROURETER: distention of ureter with urine due to obstruction.

HYPERCALCIURIA: abnormally high amounts of calcium in the urine.

HYPERPLASIA: increase in the number of cells in a tissue or organ.

HYPERTENSION: abnormally elevated blood pressure.

HYPERTONIC: having the greater osmotic pressure of two fluids.

HYPERTROPHY: excessive growth; enlargement of organ or part due to increase in size of the cells.

HYPOGASTRIC PLEXUS: a network of sympathetic nerve fibers which descend along the posterior body wall from lumbar levels to reach the pelvic organs.

HYPOTHALAMUS: a part of the brain concerned with visceral (water balance, temperature, etc.) control.

HYPOTONIC: having the lower osmolarity (concentration of ions) of two solutions.

IVP: intravenous pyelogram. An x-ray which shows the size and shape of the kidneys, ureters, and usually the bladder.

ILIAC: relating to the ilium, the broad upper wing of the pelvic bone. The term is also used to describe other structures in the region of these bones.

INANIMATE: without life.

INCONTINENCE: inability to retain a natural discharge (e.g. urine).

INTER: between.

INTERSTITIUM: space within a tissue between the cells. It is filled with connective tissue elements.

INTRA: within.

INTRAMURAL: within the wall; as where the ureter passes through the bladder wall.

INTRAVESICAL: within the bladder.

INTUSSUSCEPTION: a portion of the intestine thrust inward into another portion of the intestine.

IN VITRO: within glass—relating especially to tests performed in test tubes or outside the lining organism.

IN VIVO: within the living organism opposed to in vitro.

ISCHEMIA: lack of blood to an area of the body due to obstruction or constriction of a blood vessel.

ISOENZYME: one of multiple subunits of a protein catalyst (e.g. lactic dehydrogenase) which vary physically, chemically, or immunologically.

JAUNDICE: yellowness of skin, mucous membrane, or eyes caused by deposition of bile pigments.

JUXTA: near; next to.

KERATIN: a type of protein that forms the chemical basis of epidermis, hair, and horny-type tissue.

KINETICS: pertaining to motion, acceleration or rate of change.

LABIA MAJORA: labia (lip); majora (major). Large outer folds of tissue surrounding the vestibule. They lie lateral to the labia minora and are covered on their external surfaces with pubic hair.

LABIA MINORA: minor lips. These smaller folds surround the vestibule within the labia majora.

LABYRINTH: an intricate system of intercommunicating passages; a maze.

LAMINA/LAMINAE: a thin layer or flat plate.

LAMINA PROPRIA: connective tissue underlying an epithelium.

LATERAL: situated away from the midline.

LESION: any pathologic or traumatic structure or discontinuity of tissue.

LUMEN: the space inside a tubular or sacular structure.

LYMPHATIC CAPILLARIES: small vessels that carry excess tissue fluid (lymph) toward the heart.

LYMPHATIC TISSUE: lymphocytes; aggregations of these white blood cells are involved in the body's defense system. They attack foreign substances and bacteria.

LYMPH NODES: filters for lymph. They are small bean-shaped organs interposed in the lymphatic channels.

LYSIS: process of disintegration or dissolution of cells.

LYSOSOMES: membrane-bound cellular organelles containing hydrolytic enzymes which function in intracellular digestion. They are capable of destroying bacteria and other foreign material or their own aged organelles (autophagia).

MACRO/MICRO: large/small.

MACULA DENSA: macula (spot); densa (dense). In the kidney this refers to the distal tubule where it passes the glomerulus of origin.

MALIGNANT: disease resistant to treatment and of a fatal nature.

MEATUS: distal opening of the urethra.

MEDIAL: toward the middle of the body, or at the midline.

MEDULLA: internal, central portion of an organ.

MESANGIUM: supporting cells and matrix of the renal glomerulus.

METAPLASIA: change of one kind of tissue to another.

METASTASIS/METASTASES: a shifting from one place to another (of disease).

MICROABSCESS: localized small accumulation of pus.

MICROANGIOPATHIC HEMOLYTIC ANEMIA (MHA): fibrin clots in small vessels cause destruction of red blood cells.

MICROBIAL: pertaining to or caused by microbes (bacteria, viruses).

MICROINFARCT: tiny lesion caused by obstruction to circulation to an area.

MICTURITION: urination; the passing of urine.

MITOSIS: cell division.

MODULATE: regulation of activity in response to changing conditions.

MONONUCLEAR CELL: a cell with a single, non-lobulated nucleus; usually denotes a lymphocyte.

MONS PUBIS: pubic prominence; the fatty pad overlying the pubic symphysis of females.

MORBIDITY: illness.

MORPHOLOGY: anatomical structure or shape.

MOTILE: capable of movement.

MUCOSA: mucus secreting lining membrane of an organ. Composed of epithelium, connective tissue, and sometimes smooth muscle.

MUSCULARIS: layer of smooth muscle in the wall of hollow organs.

MYELIN FIGURES: membrane-bound residual undigested material; the by-product of intracellular digestion.

MYONEURAL JUNCTIONS: the termination of nerve endings on or near muscle.

NECROSIS: death of a cell or group of cells.

NEOPLASM: new growth; abnormal uncontrolled formation of a mass of cells or new growth of tissue (such as a tumor).

NEPHRON: functional unit of the kidney: glomerulus and tubules, but not collecting ducts.

NEUROGENIC BLADDER: malfunctioning bladder caused by interruption of, or defect in, its innervation.

NEUROTRANSMITTER: a chemical substance which transmits a nervous impulse from one nerve cell to another, or to a muscle, or to a gland.

NIDUS: nucleus; a center about which crystalization occurs.

NON–AMBULATORY: not walking.

NOSOCOMIAL INFECTION: contracted in a hospital, infirmary, or nursing home.

NOXIOUS: harmful.

OCCLUDE: close or bring together.

ORIFICE: opening or aperture.

ORTHOSTATIC HYPOTENSION: lowered blood pressure resulting from a change in position from supine to upright.

OSMOLARITY: osmotic concentration of a solution.

OSMORECEPTORS: specialized sensory endings in the hypothalamus which respond to changes in the osmolarity of blood to regulate the secretion of antidiuretic hormone.

OSMOTIC: relating to the passage of solvent of lesser concentration through a membrane to a solution of higher concentration. See solvent and solute.

OVERDISTENTION: distended beyond normal limits.

PAPILLA: the apex of the kidney medullary pyramid which projects into the minor calyx and contains the openings of the collecting ducts.

PARASYMPATHETIC NERVOUS SYSTEM: involved with conservation and restoration of energy. Nerves arise from brain stem and sacral 2, 3 and 4 levels; called craniosacral outflow.

PARASYMPATHOMIMETIC: having an action like that of the parasympathetic nervous system.

PARENCHYMA: the specific functional cells of a gland or organ as contrasted with its connective tissue framework.

PARENTERAL: introduced into the body by means other than the mouth (e.g. subcutaneous or intravenous).

PARIETAL EPITHELIUM: cells lining body cavities.

PATHOLOGY: study of the nature, cause and development of disease, and the structural and functional changes that result from disease.

PELVIC NERVES: carry parasympathetic motor fibers from S2, 3, 4 to pelvic organs, and sensory fibers from pelvic organs to the same spinal cord levels.

PENIS: male organ of copulation. It contains the urethra.

PENOSCROTAL: relating to the penis and the scrotum.

PERFUSION: passage of fluid through the vessels of an organ.

PERINEAL AREA: the area around and between the anus and genital organs.

PERINEURAL: around the nerves.

PERISTALSIS: alternate muscular contraction and relaxation of the walls of a tubular structure serving to move its contents onward.

PERISTOMAL: around the stoma.

PERITONEUM: the layer of cells lining the abdominal cavity and covering its organs.

PERITONITIS: inflammation of the peritoneum.

PERITUBULAR: peri (around), tubular (tubules).

pH: hydrogen ion concentration, or the degree of acidity or alkalinity.

PHAGOCYTE: any cell that ingests microorganisms or other cells or substances.

PHARMACEUTICALS: medications.

PHLEBITIS: inflammation of a vein, usually accompanied by clot formation.

PHYSIOLOGY: the study of the function of living organisms.

PILI: hair-like structures.

PITUITARY GLAND: produces and releases several kinds of hormones which either act directly on the body or on distant target organs.

PLEURITIC PAIN: pain arising from the inflammation of the membrane lining chest cavity and lungs.

PLEXUS: network (e.g. nerve plexus).

POLYURIA: excessive excretion of urine.

POSTGANGLIONIC: the second nerve of the two neuron chain of the autonomic nervous system with a cell body in a peripheral ganglion and an axon which reaches an effector organ. The neurotransmitter may be either acetylcholine or norepinephrine. The preganglionic neuron synapses with the postganglionic neuron.

PREGANGLIONIC: a nerve of the autonomic nervous system with a cell body in the spinal cord and an axon which is part of a peripheral nerve. The neuro-transmitter is acetylcholine.

PROSTAGLANDIN: a hormone-like substance elaborated by several tissues includ-ing the kidney medullary interstitium which causes peripheral vasodilatation and increased renal blood flow.

PROSTATE GLAND: gland the size of a chestnut surrounding the urethra immedi-ately below the bladder in the male. It secretes seminal fluid and is prone to hypertrophy in the aged.

PROTEINACEOUS: relating to, resembling, or being protein.

PROTEINURIA: excretion of protein in urine.

PROTOPLAST: a bacterial or plant cell deprived of its rigid wall.

PROXIMAL: nearest to the point of reference, in a catheter, the end nearest the inserting hand.

PUBIC BONES: a pair of pelvic bones which meet each other in front of the bladder at the symphysis pubis. They, together with the two ilia and two ischia (seat bones), make up the pelvis.

PUDENDAL NERVES: a somatic nerve with sensory and motor components aris-ing from S2,3,4 to innervate the perineal muscles, including the pelvic diaphragm and the external sphincter of the urethra.

PURULENT: containing or consisting of pus.

PYELONEPHRITIS: inflammation of the renal parenchyma and pelvis due to bacterial infection.

PYELONEPHROSIS: any disease of the pelvis of the kidney.

PYRAMID: in the kidney, the cone-shaped medullary tissue.

PYURIA: pus in the urine.

RECEPTORS: a sensory end organ, or the part of a cell membrane that combines with a chemical to cause a change in function.

RECTUM: terminal part of intestine from signoid colon to anus.

REDUNDANT: more than necessary.

REFLEX: an involuntary reaction to stimulus applied peripherally and transmitted to the central nervous system, where a motor impulse is elicited and results in the reaction.

REFLEX ARC: afferent limb (sensory fiber), nerve cell, and efferent limb (motor fiber).

RENAL: referring to the kidneys.

RENAL CORPUSCLE: glomerular tuft of capillaries and the enveloping Bowman's capsule.

RENAL FAILURE: failure of kidneys to function.

RENAL PELVIS: expanded funnel-shaped channel through which urine flows from kidney to ureter.

ROENTGENOGRAPH: X-ray.

RESECTION: surgical removal of a segment of any part of a body.

RESIDUAL: left behind; urine remaining in the bladder after voiding.

RETROGRADE: moving backward; retracing original course.

RETROPERITONEAL: behind (outside of) the peritoneum.

RIBOSOME: fine granular units within a cell that are the site of protein synthesis.

SACCULE: a small bag-like structure.

SCROTUM: fibromuscular sac which encloses the testicles.

SEBACEOUS: relating to or being a fatty material. Glands which secrete a fatty lubricant matter.

SECRETE: to make cell products and deliver them to the blood or body cavity.

SEMINAL VESICLE: diverticula of the ductus deferens which lie directly behind the bladder. They secrete a fluid rich in fructose which nourishes the sperm.

SEPTICEMIA: presence in the blood of bacterial toxins.

SEROSA: single layer of cells lining body cavities and covering internal organs. It produces a watery secretion which lubricates the movements of the organs.

SHALE: thin layer of calculous material.

SINUS: a dilated channel for blood or lymph which lacks an endothelial lining.

SINUSOID: an enlarged, irregular blood vessel, lined with endothelium.

SODIUM PUMP: an active transport system for moving sodium into and out of cells.

SOLUTE: the substance dissolved in a solution.

SOLVENT: the liquid in which a solute is dissolved.

SOMATIC: pertaining to the body wall as distinguished from the viscera.

SOMNOLENCE: sleepiness.

SPASTIC: increased tone or rigidity of a muscle.

SPHINCTER: muscle arranged around a natural body opening, which, when contracted, closes the opening.

SPINAL CORD SEGMENTS: spinal cord tissue from which arises a single pair of spinal nerves.

SPINAL SHOCK: loss of spinal reflexes after an injury, appearing in muscles and organs below the level of the injury.

SPLANCHNIC NERVES: nerves to the viscera (internal organs).

SPORICIDE: an agent that destroys spores.

SQUAMOUS: scaly or plate-like.

STAGNANT: not flowing in a current or stream.

STASIS: standing still; not moving; stoppage of flow of a fluid.

STENOSIS: narrowing or stricture.

STOMA: artificial permanent opening (as in the abdominal wall) made by surgical procedure.

STRICTURE: an abnormal narrowing of a canal, duct, or passage.

SUPRAPUBIC: above the pubic arch.

SYMBIOSIS: the living together of two dissimilar organisms for the advantage of both.

SYMPATHETIC NERVOUS SYSTEM: stimulates activities of the body which result in mobilization for emergency and expenditure of energy. The sympathetic nerves are from spinal cord segments T1 to L2, called the thoracolumbar outflow.

SYMPATHOMIMETIC: having an action like that of the sympathetic nervous system.

SYNAPSE: a gap between nerve cells, or between nerve and effector cells, through which an impulse passes from cell to cell.

SYSTEMIC: pertaining to or affecting the body as a whole.

TENESMUS: painful straining.

THRESHOLD: the degree of concentration at which a substance will be excreted by the kidneys; the value at which a stimulus will provide a sensation.

THROMBOEMBOLISM: an obstruction of a blood vessel by a dislodged clot (thrombus).

TISSUE: a mass of functionally similar cells.

TITRATE: to determine the optimum dosage by observing the effects of small changes in the amounts of medication.

TOMOGRAM: an X ray of a selected section or level of an organ or the body.

TORTUOUS: full of turns and twists.

TOXIN: a noxious or poisonous substance.

TRABECULA/TRABECULAE: a beam or column; supporting bundles of fibers; in the case of the bladder, smooth muscle fibers.

TRABECULATION: the formation of trabeculae in a part.

TRACT: a bundle of nerve fibers carrying similar information within the central nervous system; or, a passage for urine including ureter, bladder, and urethra.

TRIGONE: triangular smooth area in the base of the bladder whose apex is the urethral orifice. The ureteral orifices mark the other two angles of the trigone.

TUBULE: a small tube or canal.

TUBULOINTERSTITIAL: referring to the kidney tubules and interstitium.

TUMOR: a neoplasm; an overgrowth of tissue.

UREMIA: a toxic condition caused by failure of the kidneys to eliminate waste substances from the body.

URETER: muscular tube which conveys urine from kidney to bladder.

URETERITIS: inflammation of a ureter.

URETEROVESICAL JUNCTION: where the ureter enters the bladder.

URETHRA: passage which carries urine from bladder to exterior of the body.

URGENCY: sensation of imminent need to urinate.

URINE: the fluid excreted by the kidneys; 96 percent water, 4 percent solid matter, chiefly urea and sodium chloride.

UROPATHY: disorder of the urinary tract.

UROTHELIUM: epithelium lining the bladder; also known as transitional epithelium.

VCUG: voiding cystourethrogram. An X ray which shows the size and shape of the bladder and urethra.

VAGINA: the genital canal in the female extending from the uterus to the vestibule into which it opens.

VARIANTS: exhibiting slight differences.

VASOMOTOR: nerves that cause constriction or dilatation of blood vessels.

VEINS: blood vessels that carry blood toward the heart.

VESICAL: pertaining to the bladder.

VESICLE: a small (often microscopic) membrane-bound sac—a cellular organelle.

VESICO: pertaining to the bladder.

VESICOURETERAL REFLUX: retrograde passage of urine from bladder into ureter.

VESTIBULE: the space at the entrance to a canal.

VISCERAL EPITHELIUM: lining cells which cover an internal organ.

VOIDING: emptying the bladder.

VOLUNTARY: acting in obedience to the will.

VULVA: female external genitalia.

INDEX

Distal tubule, 6, 12, plates I-3, I-5 (*see also* Kidney, cortex, medulla)
Distention (*see* Overdistention)
Ditropan®, 146, 174, 226, 231
Diuresis (night diuresis), 46, 134, 257, 258
Diuril®, 218
Diversion (*see* Supravesical urinary diversion)
Diverticula, 62, 68, 77, 80, 115, 118, 132, 145, fig. V-8, urethral, 100 (*see also* Bladder, pathology of, Urethra, pathology of)
Dizziness (*see* Vertigo)
Donnatol®, 230, 231, 232
Double-Lumen Catheter (*see* Catheter, double lumen)
Dramamine®, 231
Drowsiness, 221, 226, 227
Drugs (*see* Pharmaceuticals)
Dry mouth, 226, 227, 231
Duvoid®, 146, 225, 231, 263
Dyscrasia, blood, 218, 221

Dysreflexia (*see* Autonomic dysreflexia)
Dyssynergia, 29, 44, 46, 62, 115, 118, 147, 225, 227, 231
Dysuria, 224

Filtration barrier (*see* Kidney, filtration barrier)
Final feeling of fullness (FFF), 238
First sensation of fullness (FSF), 238
Flagella, bacterial, 53
Flavoxate, 231
Fluid intake (*see* Diet and fluid intake)
Fluoride, 178
Fluoroscopy, 237
Flushing, 226, 249
Folic acid, 219
Food, 234 (*see also* Diet and fluid intake)
Foreign body, 225, 266
Foreskin, 128, 130 (*see also* Reproduction organs and Catheterization procedures)
Formaldehyde, 217
Freedom™, external catheter, 121 (*see also* Catheter, external)
Frequency, urinary, 224, 270
Fundus, 18, 22, 226
Furadantin, 220
Furosemide, 218, 221, 222

G

Gantanol®, 217
Gantrisin®, 217
Garamycin®, 221, 222
Garments, body support, 161–162
Gastric irritation, 220, 226
Gas sterilization (*see* Ethylene oxide)
Genes, bacterial mutations, 55
Genetic counseling, 261
Genitalia (*see* Reproductive organs)
Gentamicin, 222
Geriatric (*see* Aging)
Glanders, 60
Glaucoma, 218, 226
Glomerulus (*see* Kidney, glomerulus)
Glomerular filtration rate, GFR, 242, 248, 250, 269 (*see also* Kidney, filtration barrier)
Gout, 254
Glucose, 248
Glutaraldehyde, disinfection with, 179
Goal achievement, obstacles to, 43–44
Goals, methods for achievement, 43, 44
Goose bumps, 264
Gram stain, use for microorganism classification, 52–60, 201, 220
Gram negative (*see Gram* stain)
Gram positive (*see Gram* stain)
Grifulvin®, 219
Griseofulvin, 219
Growth rate, bacterial (*see* Bacteria, growth rate)
Guanethedine, 265

Guttman, Sir Ludwig, 131

H

Halogen, as disinfectants, 178
Hands (*see* Hand washing)
Hand washing, 127, 172–173, fig. V-3 (*see also* Catheterization procedures, and Disinfection-sterilization and Care procedures
Hay fever, 230
Headache, 219, 227, 231, 238, 240, 250, 264
Heat, disinfection and sterilization with, 175–176 (*see also* Disinfection-sterilization)
  dry, 176
  hot air treatment, 176
  incineration, 176
  moist, 175
Hematopoiesis, 43, 268
Hematuria, 63, 79, 106, 217, 224, 227, 257, 261 (*see also* Urine)
Hemoglobin, 242
Hemophilus, 221
Hepatitis, 227
Herpes, 127
Higher centers, 226 (*see also* Brain)
Hilum, 4, 6
Hiprex®, 217, 218
Hooke, Robert, 51
Hormone, 224
Hydralazine, 265
Hydration, effect on colony count, 203 (*see also* Diet and fluid intake)
Hydraulic pressure, 43 (*see also* Water hammer effect)
Hydrogen ion conc., 234
Hydrogen peroxide, disinfection with, 178
Hydronephrosis, 132, 145, 147, 151, 242, 258 (*see also* Ureter, pathology of)
Hydroureter (*see* Ureter, pathology of)
Hydroureteronephrosis (*see* Ureter, pathology of)
Hygiene (hygienic), 223, 224, 256, 261
Hypercalciuria, immobilization, 69
Hyperparathyroidism, 254
Hypertension, 226, 232, 240, 264 (*see also* Kidney, pathology of)
Hyperreflexia (*see* Autonomic dysreflexia)
Hyperreflexic bladder, 239–240
Hypotension, 226, 232

I

Ileal diversion (*see* Supravesical urinary diversion)
Ileus, 231
Imipramine, 232

Spore, bacterial, 53, 54
Sporicide, definition, 174
Squamous metaplasia, 266 (*see also* Bladder,
    pathology of)
Stagnation, 44, 235
Staphylococcus, 52, 168–169
    aureus, 60, 219, 220
    epidermidis, 61
    species, 221, 222
Stasis, 68, 252, 254 (*see also* Bladder, pathology of)
Stelazine®, 232
Sterilize, definition, 174 (*see also* Disinfection,
    sterilization)
Sterilization, gas, 179
Stimulation, 45
Stone (*see* Calculus and Obstruction)
Stoma,
    denudement, 154
    dermatitis, 154
    encrustation, 154
    pathology; bleeding, 154
    stenosis, 154
    suprapubic, 102, 103, 105, 107, 109, 111, 112
    supravesical, 151, 156, 161, 162, 163
Streak plate cultures (*see* Culture techniques)
Streptococcus, 60, 219, 221, 222
    enterococcus group 60, 220
    Lancefield classification, 60
    pyogenic group, 60
Streptomycin, 56
Stricture, 261, 262
Stroke, 225, 240, 264, 268, 271
Stuffy nose (*see* Nasal congestion)
Sudafed®, 232
Sugar, 235, 236
Sulfinpyrazone, 218, 220
Sulfonomides, 56, 217, 218–219, 256
Sunlight, 218, 220
Supersaturation, 254
Supply kits, 194–197, fig. XI-20
Suppression, 217
Supravesical urinary diversion, 45–46, 66–75, 132,
    149–165, 256, 261, 263, fig. X-1
    appliances, 156–158
        disposable, 156 fig. X-4
        reusable face plate, 156 fig. X-3
        urine collecting—leg bag, tubing, night
            drainage, 158, fig. X-5
    bladder complications, 154
    care procedures, 158, 163
        antitwist device, 160–161 fig. X-6
        body support garments, 161–162 fig. X-7
        observation, 161–162
        ostomy bag flush, 160

effect of diet and fluid intake, 155
enterostomal therapists, 163
important things to remember, 163
incidence of bacteriuria with spinal cord injury,
    167–170, tables XI-1 through 3
indications for use, 149
inherent dangers, 151–155
    calculi, 153
    infection, 67, 151–153
    peristomal pathology, 153–154
psychological problems, 155
sources of bacteriuria, 151–153 fig. X-2
types of urinary diversion, 150–151
Suppression, 217
Surgical techniques, 224, 255, 256, 262, 263, 276
Susceptibility determinations, antibiotic (*see*
    Sensitivity tests, antibiotic
Sweating, 226, 229, 231, 238, 240, 364
Swelling, 227 (*see also* Edema)

T

Tachycardia, 232
Talwin®, 231
Tarry stools, 227
Team, health, 43, 46, 121, 173, 224, 225, 234, 250, 261,
    263, 273–276
Temperature, body with spinal cord injury, 64 (*see
    also* Fever)
Tenesmus, 224
Tetracycline, 56–61, 218, 219, 220
Texas®, external catheter, 121–122
Therapist(s), occupational and physical, 275
    adaptive equipment, 276
    range of motion and exercise, 275
    role in urinary tract care, 272–280
    seat belts and clothing, 278
    supplies and literature, 276
    whirlpools, tanks and tubs, 275
Thermal death point, 175
Thermal death time, 175
Thiazide, 218
Thirst, 221
Thomas, V, 206
Thorazine®, 231
Tigan®, 231
Tiredness, 221, 227
Tissue fluid, 290
TmGl (*see* Maximal tubular excretory capacity)
TmPAH (*see* Tubular function, Maximal tubular
    excretory capacity)
Tobacco, 261
Tobramycin, 222
Tofranil®, 232